PREGNANCY

THE COMPLETE GUIDE TO EVERYTHING
YOU NEED TO KNOW ABOUT A HEALTHY
PREGNANCY THAT FITS YOUR LIFESTYLE
AND HEALS YOUR BODY AFTER
CHILDBIRTH

Pregnancy

ISBN-13: 978-1979063043

ISBN-10: 1979063044

Contents

INTRODUCTION 5

CHAPTER 1: GETTING STARTED: THINKING ABOUT GETTING PREGNANT 8
Does It Matter What a Pregnant Woman Eats? 9
50% of baby's genes come from mom and 50% come from dad. 12
Why You Can't Give to Another What You Don't Have Yourself 12
Is a Pre-Pregnancy Detox a Good Idea? 14
Foods That Affect Hormones Also Affect Fertility 14
Supplements That Fill in the Gaps 18
Good healthy digestion and elimination equal a healthy immune system. 19

CHAPTER2: EARLY PREGNANCY SYMPTOMS 21
A missed period: 22
Fatigue: 22
Abdominal bloating: 23
A frequent need to urinate: 23
Food aversion: 23
Sore Breasts: 24
Mood swings: 24
Elevated basal temperature: 25
Spotting: 25
Nausea and vomiting: 25

CHAPTER 3: THE FIRST TRIMESTER 27
Finding Out 29
Your Reaction 30
Her Reaction 31
When to Tell 31
Time to Talk: Conquering Fears, Being Supportive, and When to Say Nothing33
Dads Unite! 34
For the Mom-to-Be 34
Pregnancy Test 40
Sugar is not a nutrient-dense choice for you or your baby. 43

The liver will metabolize alcohol before it metabolizes toxins.........................45

Understanding Morning Sickness and Reducing the Symptoms 49

How Much Protein Do I Need? 51

What if I Follow a Vegan or Vegetarian Diet?..53

What if I Follow a Paleo Diet?..54

How Much Weight Gain Is Healthy..54

Keeping My Immune System Strong..55

I Am so Tired. Handling Fatigue. 56

CHAPTER 4: THE SECOND TRIMESTER...58

Staying the Course with Good Nutrition..58

Baby's Bones Are Developing: Why You Need Magnesium, Calcium, and
Antioxidants 60

Ramping Up the Calories a Little 60

Why All Calories Are Not Created Equal 61

Staying Hydrated: Water, Water, and More Water...62

CHAPTER 5: THIRD TRIMESTER-PREPARING FOR BIRTH...................................63

Avoiding Late Pregnancy Problems 65

What Happens Next If I Fail the Test? 65

Getting Blood Glucose under Control..66

Dealing with Heartburn 67

How to Avoid Constipation? 68

The Best Way to Think about Stress and Your Unborn Child..........................70

CHAPTER 6: THE FOURTH TRIMESTER: CONGRATULATIONS! YOU HAVE A NEW
BABY!...71

Bouncing Back after Birth 73

Foods that Support Lactation and Milk Production...75

How Does Diet Affect Breast Milk?...76

Taking Probiotics While I am Breastfeeding 78

Continuing Prenatal Vitamins 78

Postpartum Weight Loss...81

Why is it Important to Take Care of Yourself First Then Baby? 82

Drinking Alcohol While Breastfeeding 83

CHAPTER 7: HIGH-RISK PREGNANCY 85

Hyperemesis Gravidarum (HG): 87

Gestational Diabetes: 87

Preeclampsia: 88

Ectopic Pregnancy: 89

Placenta Previa: 90

Placental Abruption: 90

Premature Labor: 91

Social Factors 92

Teen Pregnancy 93

Bed Rest 94

CHAPTER 8: WHAT DO I NEED TO TAKE INTO HOSPITAL 95

Home Equipment Considerations 98

Other items to buy include: 101

CHAPTER 9: TAKING CARE OF HER 103

Handling the Hormones 104

You Versus the Hormones 105

Chores, Daddy Style 106

Managing Weight Gain 108

Pickles and Ice Cream 109

Pregnancy Massage 110

Pregnancy Sex 111

Exercise during Pregnancy 112

Maternity Clothes 113

CHAPTER 10: HEALING YOUR VAGINA NATURALLY 115

Early Vaginal Bleeding 116

Natural Remedies to Heal and Soothe Sore Tissue 117

When to Talk to Your Healthcare Provider: 120

Healing Vaginal Tears & Episiotomy 120

Healing Vulvovaginal Varicosities (Dilated Veins) 121

Organ Prolapse 122

Types of Prolapse: 123

Vaginal Wind 124

Is a 6-week Checkup Necessary? 125
Labs to Consider Testing Postpartum 125
Natural Relief for After Birth Pains 126
Natural Remedies to Heal Urinary Tract Infections 128
Urinary Incontinence 130
Natural Healing After a C-Section 130

CONCLUSION 133

INTRODUCTION

Thank you for purchasing this book. It is my sincere hope that it will answer all your questions about pregnancy. Becoming a mother for the first time is one of the most incredible feelings in the world. But before you get to that point, you must carry a baby for nine months.

As a woman with child, you can expect to go to the doctor often to make sure that the baby is growing as it should and ensure there are no problems that need specialist intervention. These regular doctor visits help to guarantee that you and your child are getting the best care needed. During the first trimester, you make visits to the doctor once every month in most cases. Sometimes, the doctor will want you to come in more often if you are expecting multiples or have other problems with your pregnancy. The second trimester stays pretty much the same concerning your visits, except these three months are filled with a lot of testing. In the third-trimester, things change and you are preparing to deliver your new precious bundle of joy. Your doctor will monitor you and baby closely during these last months of pregnancy.

As you go along in your pregnancy, there will be a lot of people who have such great things to tell you about what to expect. There is nothing like the pregnancy glow. You certainly are going to enjoy every single flutter of your baby inside of you. But are the nine months of pregnancy all glorious and beautiful? Most people would have you think this way, but the truth of the matter is, they are not. You are going to experience tons of weird and strange things while you are pregnant, and most of the time no one tells you about this stuff. When you are pregnant for the first time, many things happen and unless you know what to expect, you may think something is wrong. It isn't to say that pregnancy is horrible, because it is not. Being pregnant is a part of life. It is a unique time, an amazing feeling to know that you have created life and are now nourishing it into this world.

It is the purpose of this guide to provide soon-to-be mothers with the information that they need and should know while pregnant. You can learn the good, the bad and the ugly. There are so many small, silly things that come along with pregnancy, and sometimes even rather gross things. It is these things that people seem to forget to tell you.

Without further ado, continue reading to learn the secrets about pregnancy that you want to know. Learn the secrets of all the trimesters of pregnancy, as well as a few things that you should be aware of when delivering your baby and what to expect after the fact.

Pregnancy is one of the most thrilling times of your life. It is also a time in your life when amazing changes will be experienced. Now it is time to learn them all and prepare for the nine-month ride.

CHAPTER 1: GETTING STARTED: THINKING ABOUT GETTING PREGNANT

Your future child's prospects are a delicate balance between your genes and the environment. The two together have an impact on what genes get turned on and expressed and are therefore passed on to the next generation, and which genes do not. The most common factors that affect gene expression are diet, exercise, stress (environmental and emotional), and supplemental nutrition to fill in any gaps.

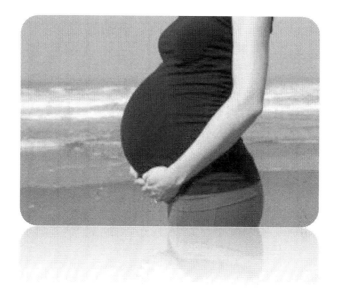

The rest of this book is designed to provide you with straightforward answers to the many questions that come to mind as you go through your journey of a balanced and beautiful pregnancy for a happy and healthy baby.

DOES IT MATTER WHAT A PREGNANT WOMAN EATS?

Yes, it matters! Studies have shown that women who have poor diets have a more challenging time in labor, and their babies run a higher risk of infections in the first year of life. Not only that, but they are also more likely to suffer from a long list of pregnancy maladies that increase the likelihood of a caesarean birth delivery.

What is also a little discouraging is that you are thrilled with the news that you are going to have a baby but you have received little or no nutritional information from your OBGYN. They are very concerned about the biometrics of pregnancy, like blood pressure, scans, weight gain, etc. However, they provide little or no input as to what the quality of the pregnancy should be, and this begins with diet, managing stress, exercise, and supplementing with whole food nutrients.

You have probably heard this statement: "It doesn't matter what I eat; the baby will just take what it needs from my body anyway." It doesn't even sound right, does it? Even if the baby takes from mom, do you want a child that survives or one that thrives? When your baby is born, it might be healthy and intelligent, but how much smarter and healthier could it have been if you had eaten properly? Another thing to consider is THE RIGHT NUTRITION MATTERS! It matters most in baby's first one thousand days, which starts at conception and goes on to the child's second birthday. What you feed yourself and your baby will define their wellness blueprint, so MAKE EVERY BITE COUNT!

We are learning more and more about the field of genetics and how the environment can affect gene expression. This area is called epigenetics.

Epigenetics means "above" or "on top of" genetics. It refers to external modifications to DNA that turn genes "on" or "off." These amendments do not change the DNA sequence, but instead, they affect how cells "read" genes.

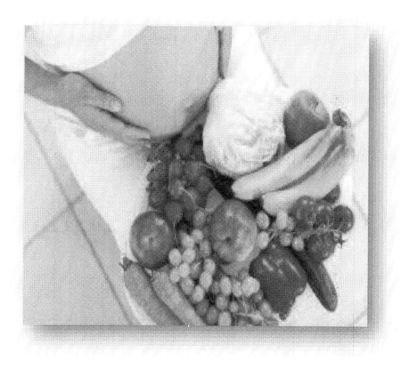

50% OF BABY'S GENES COME FROM MOM AND 50% COME FROM DAD.

It is just as important that dad has a balanced, healthy diet; keeps stress to a minimum, and exercises. Once you have conceived, we suggest parents continue their support and play an active role in ensuring that the pregnancy is sexy, loving, causes little stress, and is grounded. I am so thrilled to see more dads coming with their partners to office visits and taking a more active role in co-parenting.

WHY YOU CAN'T GIVE TO ANOTHER WHAT YOU DON'T HAVE YOURSELF

We have already briefly discussed why in a perfect and balanced world you would plan your pregnancy. Let's say you did a great job with your first pregnancy and lo and behold you are pregnant with baby number two in less than twelve months. It happens 75 percent of the time. You and your partner get a little careless or are out having too much fun and think, "Well, I am still breastfeeding, so it will be OK. I can't get pregnant anyway." Whoops! Here comes baby number two or three.

I would like you to consider that you might be a little depleted from the first pregnancy and only now starting to feel like you have a good routine in place. I hope you continued to eat well and keep stress at bay; however, I know first-time moms have a tough time. They give 150 percent of themselves to their child and do not take enough time for themselves. I see it all the time in my office. New moms come in frazzled about all kinds of things related to their first child, like the number of poops, the consistency of poops, the number of feeds, how many naps, colic, fussy, crying, birth trauma, and so on.

This behavior causes the stress level of parents to increase and therefore so does the hormone cortisol. Cortisol causes inflammation in the body and over sustained periods of time is damaging to both mom and baby. It is the case even when moms decide not to breastfeed.

Your newborn baby looks to you as its parents to see how you respond to life before he or she responds. If you are anxious and nervous, your child will be too. Continued and sustained stress increases the cravings for carbs and sugar, which then causes swings in blood sugar, resulting in changes in the microbiome (gut flora) that lays the foundation for a less-than-optimal immune system. Whew! As you can see, this cascade of events can lead to a mom and dad who are physical, nutritionally, and emotionally depleted, and most definitely not balanced.

If you want to have more than one child, consider putting the same attention and effort into the first baby as you do for baby number two, three, four, etc. Consider also that your environment affects your newborn child. Be sure to take the time to give to yourself, too. The idea is to raise a healthy family, which means parents need to take care of themselves. Be a loving and healthy example for your child/children and aim to be the best version of yourself - or better.

IS A PRE-PREGNANCY DETOX A GOOD IDEA?

As we discussed earlier in this book, in a perfect world, you would have planned your pregnancy and you and your partner would have prepared your bodies, your minds, and your spirits by doing a pre-pregnancy detox.

FOODS THAT AFFECT HORMONES ALSO AFFECT FERTILITY

The most common foods that influence productivity are those you are sensitive to and that cause a reaction in your body.

You could have a full-blown reaction, or it could be something subtle like a rash, runny nose, or brain fog. You could be sensitive to gluten, soy, dairy, peanuts, and chocolate. Foods you are sensitive to are those that create an inflammatory response in the body and therefore affect the gut lining and the microbiome (gut flora). If you continue to consume foods you are sensitive to, over time you could potentially develop an autoimmune-type response, which will typically show up in an endocrine organ.

One example is the thyroid, and the autoimmune diagnosis is called Hashimoto's thyroiditis. A thyroid that is not functioning well has a cascade type effect on the other glands in the endocrine system, and therefore affects the reproductive organs and fertility.

Everything you eat is beneficial, neutral, or damaging to your microbiome (gut flora); and therefore, foods can have a positive, negative, or neutral effect on your gene expression.

The most common foods that account for 75 percent of all food sensitivity reactions are:

- Wheat and gluten containing foods
- Corn
- Soy
- Processed cow dairy
- Eggs
- Peanuts

We also suggest that you reduce your toxic load as it relates to bath and body products, cleaning products, and air fresheners. These products contain xenoestrogens, which mimic the effects of estrogen, which, in turn, can affect normal hormonal function.

We have talked about food, environmental toxins, and health challenges and how these factors can affect fertility. Here are a few other things to consider:

- Is your diet low in good-quality protein?
- Are you eating enough healthy high-quality fats?

- Are you skipping meals and therefore have low blood sugar (hypoglycemia) tendencies? A little sugar causes a spike in cortisol, which affects your hormone levels.
- High blood sugar can also have an impact. If you are overweight and eating too many simple carbohydrates, it is time to re-evaluate your diet.
- Are you under high stress? Take a step back and look at your life and see where you can make some changes. Consider incorporating meditation or some other calming techniques.
- Are you getting enough healthy minerals in your diet? Increasing your veggies is a good natural way to supplement minerals. Adding a green drink also adds big value.

Knowing this, imagine the steps the body must take to convert a food or substance with a lot of chemicals or a ton of preservatives, with names you cannot pronounce, into energy. Also, imagine how much extra work the liver must do to eliminate these toxins from so-called foods! These foods have little or no nutritional value, yet they require a ton of energy.

What Is Best for My Family and Me?

There is a lot of information out there about what is right and what is not so great surrounding the topic of pregnancy and birth. In fact, you can expect more than your fair share of advice. Random strangers will feel the need to stop you and give their sage advice. It can all be overwhelming, and this is where you need to tap into what is uniquely you.

You and your partner bring your entire selves to the process of having a balanced and beautiful pregnancy and a happy, healthy baby. It is the sum of your combined experiences, feelings, genes, emotions, etc., that go into making this baby. What is right for one couple might not be right for you.

One of the biggest challenges today is that there is too much information "out there" and not enough grounded in the natural process of things. Pregnancy and birth is a "natural process" that should be filled with positivity and hope, not worry and fear.

The process of birth can be overwhelming; and before you know it, you are concentrating on all the things that could go wrong. Focusing on all the risks and none of the rewards, you can miss the experience. All these stress transfers to your unborn child, which is not good for the baby or you. Trust your body: it was meant to be able to do this.

SUPPLEMENTS THAT FILL IN THE GAPS

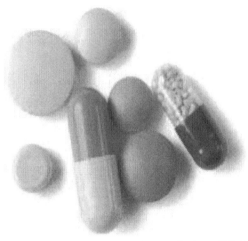

The following supplements are intended to fill in the gaps and not to make up for a poor diet. We are assuming you are doing a good job of eating your nutrients.

Probiotics

Probiotics provide our digestive system with healthy bacteria, enabling optimal immune function.

If you have taken antibiotics during your life, then you know that while antibiotics do their job and kill off the bad bugs, they also kill off the real bugs. The gut microbiome can become unbalanced, and this can lead to digestive distress, malabsorption of nutrients, skin issues, allergies, and various other immune problems. Taking a probiotic is about putting the good bugs back into the digestive tract and creating balance.

GOOD HEALTHY DIGESTION AND ELIMINATION EQUAL A HEALTHY IMMUNE SYSTEM.

A healthy immune system is good for both mom and baby. The best time to start your probiotic is pre-conception.

Omega-3 Fatty Acids

Healthy fats also reduce inflammation, regulate blood sugar, maintain cardiovascular health, and improve immune function. Looking for a good source is important.

Many of the big chain store products are heat processed and may be rancid, causing increased inflammation instead of calming it down. Look for cold-pressed sources from places like Norway. With these products, you can be sure the supplement is super clean and does not contain mercury. Krill oil is also an excellent source of omega-3 fatty acids. If you are vegan or vegetarian, you can add flax seed oil, chia seeds, hemp seeds, and black currant oil to your supplement plan. While not an omega-3, evening primrose oil has been used for hundreds of years to address inflammatory conditions and has a rich source of anti-inflammatory omega-6 (GLA).

Vitamin D3

Vitamin D3 is essential for healthy teeth and strong bones. Vitamin D helps with the absorption of calcium and is of particular importance during pregnancy. If your levels are low, less than 40 ng/ml (the functional range is 40–80 ng/ml), then you need to supplement to bring the levels up.

B12

B12 works with folate to help support the proper fetal development and prevent neural tube defects. We talked about B12 under "What Additional Tests I should consider and why?"

CHAPTER2: EARLY PREGNANCY SYMPTOMS

There are a variety of symptoms you may experience during early pregnancy. Not all women experience the same ones, and they can differ with successive pregnancies. Some can appear when you have missed a period, others not for a few weeks. Here are a few:

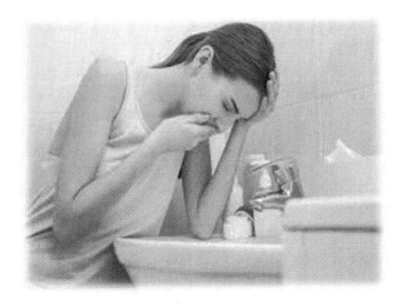

A MISSED PERIOD:

Women that have regular periods, but then miss one may do a pregnancy test before any other symptoms occur. For others with irregular periods, the first inkling they might be pregnant could be breast tenderness, nausea or needing the loo more often!

FATIGUE:

You might not just feel sleepy; you may be exhausted! Although no one is sure, it may be the increase of the hormone progesterone that makes you feel tired. Obviously, if you need to wee more often and you feel sick, this can add to the tiredness. Women usually start to have more energy once into the second trimester. Tiredness will usually return in late pregnancy when the weight of the baby makes it harder for you to get a good night's sleep.

ABDOMINAL BLOATING:

As with a period, the hormones associated with early pregnancy can make you feel bloated. So, even though there is no outward sign of gestation, your clothes may feel a little tight.

A FREQUENT NEED TO URINATE:

Hormonal changes in pregnancy mean that the blood flow to your kidneys increases. It means your bladder fills more quickly, which in turn makes you pee more often! This frequent need to wee increases later in pregnancy, when the baby's weight puts more pressure on your bladder.

FOOD AVERSION:

It can be common for women in early pregnancy to feel

nauseated when confronted with certain smells e.g. coffee, spicy food. It can often be things that you enjoyed before pregnancy. Strong smells may even make you want to gag. Although experts do not know for certain why this occurs, it may be due to the increasing amount of estrogen in your system.

SORE BREASTS:

Rising hormone levels can cause sensitive swollen breasts, again like before a period. It should ease after your first trimester, as your body becomes more used to the hormonal changes

MOOD SWINGS:

These are common in early pregnancy and are due to hormone changes that affect the chemical messengers in your brain. Some mums-to-be may feel a positive effect; others may feel depressed or anxious. If you are finding it hard to cope, make sure to contact your healthcare provider immediately.

ELEVATED BASAL TEMPERATURE:

Your basal temperature is the lowest measurement of your body's temperature when taken first thing in the morning. Some women chart their temperature, to establish when they are due to ovulate, and therefore more likely to conceive. If it remains high for over two weeks, then you are likely pregnant.

SPOTTING:

It is natural to feel concerned if after wanting to be pregnant, you then see bleeding. If the bleeding is severe, accompanied by pain, or you just need reassurance, contact your midwife or doctor.

NAUSEA AND VOMITING:

Commonly known as "morning sickness," It usually starts at about eight weeks into pregnancy; but for some women, it can appear as early as two weeks. It can also occur any time of day or night. Nausea will usually begin to ease by the start of the second trimester. Some of the following may mean you are at more risk of developing nausea and vomiting.

- A first pregnancy.
- Multiple pregnancy, e.g. twins or triplets.

- Nausea and vomiting in a previous pregnancy.
- A family history of nausea and vomiting in gestation. For example, if your mum experienced morning sickness carrying you, you may find you will too!
- If you have experienced nausea when using contraceptives that contain estrogen.
- If you suffer from motion sickness; for example, traveling in a car.
- Being obese with a body mass index (BMI) of 30 or more.
- Stress.

CHAPTER 3: THE FIRST TRIMESTER

The first quarter is a good time for both of you to mentally prepare yourselves and begin adjusting to your new lives as parents. The BMP will feel changes in the body as pregnancy hormones start to take effect. The uterus will grow during this time, up to the size of a grapefruit in preparation for the baby's growth. This little human comes complete with the DNA blueprint to form all his or her body parts, from the halo atop her head all the way down to her toes. This baby will grow faster than your student loans: between day one and the ninth week of growth, the little-fertilized embryo will grow to about an inch long. While every woman and every pregnancy are different, your BMP may begin to experience symptoms, including heartburn, headaches, mood swings, and morning sickness.

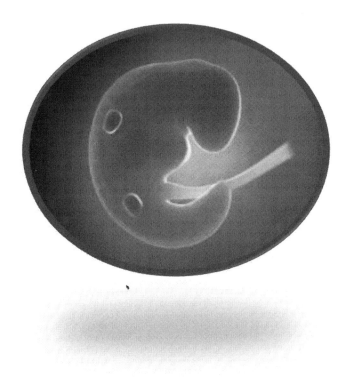

Dad, you will feel pretty good. The same, in fact. The best ways to do this will be to get informed, be supportive, and most of all, be patient. Oh, and if she gets a severe case of morning sickness, hold her hair while she gets sick.

When the pregnancy test stick turns blue, the light to fatherhood goes green. It's something you've dreamed about most of your life. You and your buddies stayed up late, wearing your purple pajamas, having tickle fights, and talking endlessly about your dreams of parenthood.

Or maybe not.

In any case, the time to prove yourself as a superior über-parent is fast approaching. If this book is in your hand, you're either an expectant father or intentionally headed in that direction.

FINDING OUT

She suspects she's pregnant. She misses her period, or else she's charting her ovulation cycle, and she knows you've got a good chance of getting good news. In a rush of excitement, she'll start the pregnancy testing game. Set aside $50 or more for this excellent match. If she sends you to the store to pick up the pregnancy test kit, I recommend buying the economy pack.

Be advised, even if she gets a positive test, she will take several more tests just to be sure — hence the budgetary concern. It means multiple trips to the pharmacy for you and lots of laser-guided urine attacks on testing sticks for your BMP. Don't be frustrated. This ritual opens the doorway to fatherhood. And don't discount the possibility of a real celebration between the two of you.

If all goes well, at some point you'll get the good news: she's pregnant! Way to go, champ. Now you feel that different emotion that bonds all first-time fathers together.

Your internal monologue asks if you're up to the challenge.

"No worries," you think to yourself. "I have nine months before I need to be concerned about this. Besides, my beautiful mother-to-be will be taking care of most of it."

YOUR REACTION

Your first reaction may be to pop the cork, open some wine, or shake a martini. Um, slow down there. Put the olives and vermouth away. Remember that the newly anointed mother of your child cannot drink alcohol. Unless she is kind enough to grant permission, you should refrain as a gesture of solidarity. You know, it's like you're saying, "Yep, we're in this thing together."

While you sip sparkling grape juice and reminisce about New Year's Eve when you were twelve, you'll probably wonder how long you have to get ready before the stork shows up. Traditionally, the number is forty weeks from the date of her last period. You'll get an "official" due date from the doctor based on information she gives him about her cycle, anything she knows about her ovulation, and other factors; but remember, it's only an estimate. In other words, don't get your firstborn's due date tattooed on your shoulder before the actual birth.

You may feel pressure begin to build as you realize that fatherhood is just around the corner. You may even experience pure, unadulterated fear. You will soon be a father and have all the responsibility that it entails.

A strange phenomenon occurs when you have a whole bunch

of stressful, exhausting days in a row, and you think about changing your name to Juan Valdez and hopping the next plane to Parts Unknown, South America, but then your child will do something that makes it all seem worthwhile. Maybe it's a simple smile or the way he greets you with a huge smile right when you arrive home from work. Maybe it's the first time you hear your child call you "Daddy." In ways both small and large, this baby will affect you in ways you can't predict.

HER REACTION

Like most men most of the time, you'll be in touch with your feelings, but what about your BMP? She will most likely feel a hundred emotions at once. You are excited and thinking, "This 's great." She is starting there and then wondering how far she'll get. Maybe she's feeling some fear at the thought of giving birth, hopeful that you are excited, and worried about labor pain. See what I mean? You can see how things are much different in BMP-world than for you and your simple caveman brain. In fact, she's already thinking.

WHEN TO TELL

After conversing with some pregnancy veterans, I put together this plan for your consideration:

First Month

Keep it on the down low (unless that means what my wife told me Oprah said it means — then forget I used this phrasing!). The two of you can exchange knowing glances and have your little secret all to yourselves. Many people will go ahead and let their close family know, but be warned: some grandparents-to-be can be, well, intense. They can pick a name, buy clothes for the baby, and help her apply to college all while you're still looking at the plus sign on the pregnancy test stick. The whole thing escalates to a new level. Just make sure the grandparents know before the public as a whole. If they're the last to know, they may never forgive you, and surely you'll need them to help out in the future.

Second Month

Trial and error have proven the best way to go here. You can each tell one friend, as friends can share in your excitement, and you'll have someone new to discuss this grand news with. Yes, this is more for her benefit, as most guys will exchange fist bumps and then get back to sports or the stock market.

Third Month

It's about time to release the hounds. Tweet, Facebook, email--go for it all as long as you both agree to it. If you want to, have a baby shower More on that later. But back to some of the more creative methods to alert friends and family of your BMP's condition:

1. Feeling nostalgic? Plaster "Baby on Board" stickers all over your house and car.
2. Give your parents and in-laws a "World's #1 Grandparent" T-shirt, and watch them smile.
3. Even the dimmest family members will get it when you play them with copies of the ultrasound photo, email them the website link or wrap up a printout in a gift box.

There is also the matter of the family hierarchy, something you'll need to consider to prevent hurt feelings on the part of friends or family.

TIME TO TALK: CONQUERING FEARS, BEING SUPPORTIVE, AND WHEN TO SAY NOTHING

Men are men. This straightforward and absurd statement can be exhaustively analyzed until your head spins, and I plan to do just that. Men, you and I are simply people: the stereotypical man. Some of the expectations that come with being the stereotypical ma: he is indestructible, is weakened only by kryptonite, can fly, and is a poor communicator.

We tend to keep things, such as problems or concerns we're having, to ourselves. Our role upon entering manhood initiation was to carry all the burdens given to us and never discuss our feelings. Ever. So, because communication is such an important part of any adult relationship, especially including ones involving a baby, we need some substantial help from the women in our lives.

DADS UNITE!

Staying informed is one thing women execute better than we do. They organize and analyze. They had so much information available targeted at them; it would be hard for any female with an Internet connection not to be a well-informed pregnant lady. But I was thinking of what old dads (like me) would tell a newly-minted pregnant mother (your BMP) about how to help the newest daddy on the block (you) during this time of adjustment for everyone. See if you can get her to read this section. Try leaving the book open on her pillow or telling her you to want to swap pregnancy books. While you're fake-reading her book, watch her read this one and see her reaction. If this section gets you into trouble, you can always claim you haven't read this far and disagree with everything I've written.

FOR THE MOM-TO-BE

Here are some things you may have trouble saying to your BMP; I'm going to say them for you:

He Feels Left Out in the Cold
The whole baby thing is taking place inside the mother, and physically, she's undergoing the most changes. But with

everything so focused on mommy, dad sometimes can feel like the sperm donation was the essential part for him to play. Doctor's visits, admiring the baby bump — of course, that's where most of the focus will be. But many of these items do not directly involve your man, and they're not natural activities that he's going to dive right into. It can all add up to a dad who isn't feeling connected to the baby right up through the whole birth process.

This Pregnant Woman is Difficult to Deal With

There, I said it. And I'm not taking it back. Dealing with a pregnant woman can be like dealing with an unhappy person with a multiple-personality disorder. It seems like there are many personalities in there and we can't switch gears fast enough to keep up. To hang tough, your guy needs to know that the woman he loves is in there somewhere. How can you show that? The easiest answer is to do something the two of you used to do together. But don't be afraid to break away from the herd. You two are beginning an entirely new type of relationship, and you may want to dream up a new activity accordingly. Have dinner and declare the conversation to be baby-free. Although most people look at children as the glue in a family, it's a healthy relationship between the parents that matters most. Keep up the required maintenance on your relationship, and make sure all the parts are running smoothly. (Yes, I just compared your relationship to a car.) Point your man to websites dedicated to pregnant women, where he'll discover useful information (as well as how the idea that pregnant women can say or ask just about anything from us gets perpetuated).

He Gets the Blues Too

Ladies, if you've done your homework, you know the risk of depression that women can face around pregnancy and parenthood. Men are in danger as well. A new study shows that up to 15 percent of men suffer from postpartum depression. And that's only the number of wimps who are willing to admit it. Between the emotional and financial stress and friends and family focusing on the glowing mom or the arriving baby, dad is out of the spotlight.

Let's not forget that post-birth depression is not only for women. Finally, something we can share! Unfortunately, after Junior comes home, both mom and dad can feel overloaded, unsure, and exhausted. Despite what the pharmaceutical industry says, no magic pill can make it pass (if you disagree, ignore my advice and see a doctor). But talking it out (I know, we men hate to do this) and trying to stay as rested and healthy as possible are good first lines of defense.

Share with Your Man

A note to women: he's not used to sharing you. He's used to getting most of your love and attention, and whenever possible, a little extra something-something from you. On a personal level, he wants to know he's still your special guy. He is losing your attention pre-birth, and he's sure to lose it post-birth. So be creative and spend some time just with him. Give him a week where he's the only one who gets to touch the baby bump. Be flexible and take him to Vegas. Okay, maybe that's going too far. But you need to work together to keep each other happy.

He's worried because he knows that the new family member not only takes away some of your time and attention but also affects your sex life.

Please take note: sex is essential to most men. Can this be stressed enough? Don't get me wrong; your husband will enjoy having a baby and will be excited. It's just that part of his relationship with you has this most enjoyable unique form of interaction. So please don't forget about it, because he didn't.

Give Me a T!

Remember all those things that pregnant women need to do before their guilt overwhelms them — like eat healthier and exercise? Make him go along with you. Everything is easier with a friend; and if you and your man are creating a child together, you at least qualify as friends and will remain so. Oh, and you're giving me a T, as in T-E-A-M, because you're in this together and need to help each other out. You will need each other to play different roles through this new challenge. Some days you'll need to motivate each other, sometimes you'll need to complain to each other, and sometimes you'll just need to play straight up "boss and secretary" with each other. But whatever each day brings, you'll always need each other.

Make Him Talk

I can't believe I'm saying this after all those times when I didn't feel like talking about something. But it has to be done. Since guys don't call each other up and chit-chat about how being a father makes them feel or about their fears (just so you know, we have none), it's up to you, a VIP BMP, to pull this stuff out of your man and make him discuss it. Because, hey, he's got worries too, or at least he will when he stops and realizes what having a baby means to your lives. So, unless you have the rare man who begins a conversation with, "Hey, honey, I have some concerns about what having a baby together will mean to our relationship and our lives together," he may need you to get the ball rolling.

Be Patient: Remember That He Doesn't Always Plan Things Out

This may be an understatement. Most men certainly don't think about our plan, and then think again about our plan, and then plan to further plan. You, your BMP, may have read three articles and changed your opinion on an issue twice before you ask him. He usually thinks for about two to three seconds and gives you his best guess. So, please work with him on these conversations and try to avoid ambushing him with questions like, "What will we do if our new daughter has trouble making friends with other children?" Ummm, he doesn't know. And he hasn't thought about it, but it doesn't mean he doesn't care.

Change He Can Believe in

It can make him feel slightly less than manly and these activities can also make him late for his facial and body waxing. So, while he needs to work on being more sensitive to the myriad changes you're experiencing, his big lumbering male ego will need a tune-up as well.

Promises, Promises

But you can work something out to ensure that you do fun and unique things together after Junior becomes part of the family. Leave your man a note with your perfume on it, with only a date, and no explanation. Send a calendar reminder to his e-mail or electronic calendar that says, "Human Resources Training: Sexual Harassment," and then show him how to break all the policies in the employee handbook. It might just start a playful back and forth that will keep the relationship fun for everyone.

Men, bonding with your woman should be comfortable enough. You've already explored one form of bonding to get here. But now it's time to bond in more creative, yet less orgasmic ways.

Talk about what these life changes are going to mean for both of you. Discuss plans for your child after her birth. Make it clear to your BMP that you still expect a hot meal and foot rub upon your arrival home from work. These are the important things that will ease the changes that are sure to happen.

Building a relationship with your unseen child can feel a little strange. Suggested methods include massaging your BMP's belly while talking to your creation.

If it feels slightly unnatural to stare into your BMP's navel and tell the fuzz lingering in there how your day went, but don't worry. It's all part of the birthing process. Just come up with something you can accept that will begin forming that bond between you and your child. (Do I have any suggestions? I thought you'd never ask!)

Here are a few more concrete activities that will help you build that bond:

- Doctor visits. There are a lot of these, but try to think of them as the time you're taking together to check on Junior's health and to stay informed about what's going on. See Chapter 3 for more about this.
- Ultrasound. It is a major bonding moment for a lot of people. You will confirm that all the fingers and toes are there and learn the sex of your child if you desire. If you want some fun, check around the area to see if 3-D ultrasound is available. Reports are that the details are stunning — you can see exactly what your child is doing in there and what he looks like.
- Discussing Junior's future. It seems far-fetched to talk about where your baby may attend college, but an excellent discussion of your child's future can drift into what might be referred to as "slightly optimistic" territory. Dream a little dream together and let it bring you closer together emotionally. If it does the same physically, so much the better.

PREGNANCY TEST

Many home pregnancy tests are not sensitive enough to detect you are pregnant until approximately a week after you've missed a period. If it shows a negative result, wait a few days and try again. Looking after your health is vital, even if you don't have a positive effect yet.

When is the right time to take a pregnancy test?

There are different pregnancy tests available, depending on the timing of conception and your preference; There is the classic urine test and a blood test. The hormone present in your body during pregnancy is called human chorionic gonadotrophin (hCG).

If you think you are pregnant but received a negative result on your home pregnancy test, don't worry. False-negatives can occur due to a variety of factors: The urine was too dilute to detect hCG, the test was done incorrectly, or you tested too soon, or home pregnancy test has passed its use by date. Fertility medication or other drugs containing hCG can interfere with home pregnancy tests. However, other medicines, such as antibiotics or birth control pills shouldn't.

It is rare, but false-positives do occur and can be due to blood or protein being present in your urine. Certain drugs, such as anticonvulsants or tranquilizers can also cause false-positive test results.

Whether you have received a positive or negative result with a home pregnancy test, it is always best to seek the advice of a medical professional as soon as possible.

Pregnancy Due Date

How can you calculate your baby's due date? Women do not have same menstrual cycles; and if you have irregular periods, your due date may be difficult to pinpoint. However, if you have a regular menstrual cycle of 28 days, you can estimate a due date by adding 280 days (nine months, seven days) to the first day of your last period. Please remember this is not always 100% accurate and should be taken as an estimate only.

It may seem strange, as it means you are officially pregnant before you conceive! Only 5% of babies are born on their due date. 80% of women deliver somewhere between 37 and 42 weeks, which means approximately 15% are premature. Although there may not always be an obvious reason, there are certain risk factors that suggest you may go into labor early, e.g. multiple pregnancies, infection.

If you are a woman with irregular periods, how can you determine your due date? First, if you can remember the date of your last menstrual cycle, you can still use the calculation above. Another way for a midwife to estimate your baby's due date is to palpate your abdomen. They assess the fundal height: this is the top of the uterus (which reaches your navel at around 20 weeks.) An ultrasound scan can also be performed to determine your expected due date if other methods have not worked or your midwife wants to confirm it.

A cesarean section is an alternate way to give birth, and your due date may not be the only thing to consider if one is required. They are usually scheduled no sooner than seven days before your due date. However, and whenever your baby is born, enjoy the moment. Many women would tell you that children usually come when they are ready; remember a due date is just an estimate!

Antenatal Screening

Screening is an important part of pregnancy. When to test and what tests to have are important questions; whether you are pregnant with your first child or been pregnant before, any testing can be nerve-wracking. Antenatal screening is carried out in all three trimesters. Every test is important, as they help assess both you and your baby's health, at different stages of your journey.

Hospitals in the UK offer all pregnant women at least two ultrasound scans during pregnancy. There are no known risks to either you or your baby, but it is important to make sure you have all the facts before having an ultrasound. If you choose not to go ahead, your choice will be respected, and you can continue with all other aspects of antenatal screening. Talk to you midwife/doctor about your concerns.

SUGAR IS NOT A NUTRIENT-DENSE CHOICE FOR YOU OR YOUR BABY.

Sugar and Sugar Substitutes

What you eat, your baby eats. Sugary snacks and foods have no nutritional value and lead to blood sugar swings, which have an enormous impact on fetal development. Keeping blood sugar stable will help you avoid nausea, **morning sickness**, problems with **gestational diabetes**, anxiety, cloudiness, irritability, and the jitters.

Trans Fats and Vegetable Oils

We discuss this and olive oil fraud under "Good Fats," if you need to review it.

Alcohol, Drugs, and Cigarettes

It is evident; however, if you need to take drugs or have a health concern, please check in with your OBGYN. It would also be worth your time to consult a wellness practitioner to help you with the cause resolution for what ails you.

What about a glass of wine? Your body goes through a myriad of hormonal changes during pregnancy, and they affect the entire endocrine system. In fact, the liver is an endocrine organ, so using things metabolized by it during pregnancy (like alcohol and many drugs) puts extra stress on this vital organ.

THE LIVER WILL METABOLIZE ALCOHOL BEFORE IT METABOLIZES TOXINS

Soft Drinks

If you can, wean yourself off of soft drinks before pregnancy and never choose to drink them again. If you decide to drink them postpartum, you will have a tough time keeping your kids away from them. They see what you and hubby drink and eat, and they will want what you consume. The cycle of poor diet and unhealthy behaviors will keep on perpetuating itself.

What about Coffee and Other Drinks?

There are lots of conflicting opinions on what is safe.

Here is what we know: Caffeine blocks the absorption of iron and raises your cortisol levels, which then impacts the adrenal glands. There is a lot of discussion out there about coffee. Here's how you need to think about it. Coffee often raises cortisol levels in the body. Cortisol is the stress-handling hormone secreted by the adrenal glands in response to stress.

Due to the hormonal changes taking place during pregnancy, it is vital that the adrenal glands are strong and weight be kept to a minimum. Pregnancy is stressful, and the adrenals need to be strong to have the healthy pregnancy you want.

High cortisol has an impact on energy levels, blood sugar

levels, and much more. If you do choose to have coffee, we suggest you have only one cup a day and decide to enjoy it with coconut milk, goat milk, full-fat organic milk, or half and a half. The fat in the coffee will slow the release of caffeine into the body. We also suggest that you keep an eye on your iron levels.

Other Drinks

We are firmly suggest that you avoid sugary drinks like sodas and alcohol. Stick to plain water with a spritz of lemon in it. Protein shakes are also a very good idea. For the Ultimate Protein Shake recipe go to page 116.

High Mercury Fish

Avoid tuna, swordfish, and shark, as they are large fish and accumulate mercury. Mercury is a toxic metal and it impacts brain function. 'Nuff said.

Raw Seafood

It is best to avoid raw seafood, including fresh sushi, due to possible complications from parasites and worms.

Soft Cheeses

Soft cheeses are made with unpasteurized milk that may harbor listeria bacteria, which can be life-threatening for mom and her unborn baby.

Raw Eggs

It is best to avoid raw eggs due to the possibility of salmonella bacteria. Say no to homemade Caesar dressing, hollandaise sauce and mayonnaise.

Mixed Bag

- Deli meats and hot dogs: They contain a myriad of chemicals known to contain listeria bacteria.
- Chinese food: Often it contains MSG, an excitotoxin very damaging to the body and, more importantly, the brain.
- Soy: If you choose to eat soy look for fermented organic sources. It is pro-estrogenic and can mimic estrogen and upset the hormonal balance of the body. The other concern with soy is that it is highly processed and genetically modified (GMO).
- Peanuts: Peanuts are a high-risk food and allergen and known to contain mold. Peanuts are not nuts; they are legumes. Can peanuts be healthy? Yes, they can be if you buy high-quality, organic peanuts like Valencia peanuts and you get plenty of omega-3 fats in your diet to offset the high amount of omega-6 fat found in them.
- Dairy: Choose organic sources from grass-fed cows. Of particular note: The primary protein in cow's milk is casein, which is hard for the body to digest. Pasteurization transforms lactose found in milk into beta-lactose sugar, which causes rapid absorption, spikes blood sugar, and therefore increases

insulin. Remember, cow dairy is highly processed; therefore, choose organic pasture-raised raw sources.

- The dangerous parts of the milk proteins are only present in minimal amounts in butter, and they are enzymatically modified during the butter pasteurization process. For this reason, butter can be a good choice as fat.

Herbal tea: We suggest you consume herbal tea with caution. There is a lot of conflicting data about what herbs are and are not safe for pregnant moms. The other question is the quality of the herbal products available. Are you sure of the source?

Most herbs are contra-indicated for pregnant and lactating moms; however, some midwives suggest raspberry leaf tea to help with delivery. I would enjoy fresh herbs like parsley, ginger, and rosemary in moderation. Of particular note: Green tea increases the need for folic acid. So, if you want to have green tea, make sure you are getting adequate folic acid in its active form: folate.

UNDERSTANDING MORNING SICKNESS AND REDUCING THE SYMPTOMS

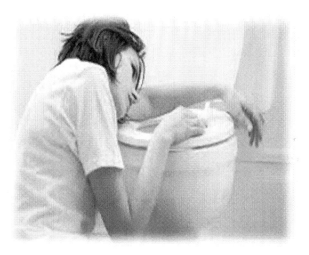

Morning sickness is one of the ways a woman's body protects baby from the toxins in food. Toxins make everyone sick, and women who are pregnant are much more sensitive to them, particularly in the first ten to twelve weeks of pregnancy.

The change in your hormones cause fluctuations in the entire endocrine system, and women who experience other endocrine challenges or a compromised digestive track are often more likely to have problems with morning sickness.

Toxins make everyone sick, and pregnant women are much more sensitive.

Here's another way to think about morning sickness: You have found out that you are pregnant, so wanting to make sure you have a healthy baby, you suddenly cut out a bunch of foods and drinks from your diet.

If they were foods and drinks you were consuming on a regular basis (an example would be coffee), the body would go through a detox process. So, not only are you dealing with changes in hormones, but you are also going through a mild to moderate detoxification. If your liver function is perfect, then you might have a slight headache and be fine. If your liver does not work optimally, then you will probably struggle with nausea and fatigue. This mechanism is there to protect your baby while your body rids itself of toxins.

The first twelve weeks are crucial in early development when cell division is very rapid. By the end of twelve weeks, your baby is fully formed. If you are craving things like ice or metals, that is another story. You should check in with your practitioner because there could be a more serious issue going on. Here are some other possibilities that could be the cause of your nausea and morning sickness.

Adrenal stress: If the adrenals are weak, the changes that occur during the early stages of pregnancy can cause morning sickness. We have had success in treating and supporting the adrenal glands. Stressors to the adrenal glands could be physical, emotional, or nutritional. What we mean is too little or too much in either one of these areas.

Other hormonal challenges: The endocrine organs work on an active and negative feedback system. If you have dysfunction in another endocrine organ, that could have an impact on morning sickness. Examples would be PCOS (polycystic ovarian syndrome), blood sugar challenges like hypoglycemia or insulin resistance, uterine fibroids, and a history of PMS. Not enough sleep can cause disruption; so can thyroid difficulties and liver and gallbladder dysfunction. If you know you have endocrine problems, a P21 program should be part of your plan.

If you do feel nauseous, try to eat protein and fat first and not simple carbs. Try to eat small meals often and pay attention to triggers. For some people, ginger is helpful as it aids in digestion and neutralizes the acids that can cause nausea and vomiting.

HOW MUCH PROTEIN DO I NEED?

Pregnant women need between 80-90 grams of protein a day for a healthy pregnancy. Proteins provide the essential amino acids needed to build a healthy human. Not enough protein and the body will take it from muscle, which will deplete muscle mass; too much will put a strain on the kidneys and liver.

The body does not store amino acids. Therefore, we suggest that you aim for 25 grams per meal and then add a high protein snack like organic raw or dry roasted nuts to hit your daily target. To help you understand what 80 grams of protein should look like, consider the following table:

PROTEIN TYPE	MEASUREMENTS	GRAMS
Lean Grass Fed Beef	6 oz.	54 grams
Turkey	6 oz.	51 grams
Chicken, dark	6 oz.	49 grams
Chicken, white	6 oz.	38 grams
Fish	3 oz.	22 grams
Almonds	1 cup	20 grams
Peas	1 cup	10 grams
Black Beans	1 cup	15 grams
Hummus	1 cup	12 grams
Lentils	1 cup	18 grams
Oatmeal	1 cup	11 grams
Quinoa	1 cup	8 grams
Plain Greek Yogurt	1 cup	10 grams
Spinach, cooked	1 cup	5 grams
Broccoli	1 cup	4 grams
Pumpkin Seeds	1oz	5 grams
Peanut Butter	1oz	7 grams
Tempeh	1oz	5 grams
Chia Seeds	1 teaspoon	3 grams
Spirulina	1 teaspoon	2 grams
Egg	One	6 grams

WHAT IF I FOLLOW A VEGAN OR VEGETARIAN DIET?

Here are some of the pitfalls we see when moms follow a vegan and vegetarian diet. Moms tend to consume:

Vegetarian and vegan moms tend to consume too much soy protein, which for some can contribute to thyroid problems. We discussed how the endocrine system is linked and how one gland can affect another. The increase and shift in hormones during pregnancy can affect the thyroid. Soy has also been identified as an allergenic food, and there is lots of speculation as to the genetic modification of this food. With that being said, stick with organic and fermented sources of soy like tempeh, miso, and tamari.

Another challenge we see for vegan and veggie moms is keeping up with the amount of suggested protein their growing baby needs. Please check out the protein guide located page 52 to help ensure you are getting a variety of foods in adequate amounts.

We also suggest you consume plenty of healthy fats, deeply pigmented veggies, nuts, and seeds. Women who typically follow a vegan or vegetarian diet often struggle to keep their blood sugar in a healthy range. Again, saying it twice, if you are a vegan or vegetarian mom, I strongly encourage you to make sure you get plenty of healthy fat, lots of nutrient dense, colorful veggies, and high-quality protein.

WHAT IF I FOLLOW A PALEO DIET?

Here are some of the pitfalls we see when moms follow a strict Paleo diet: moms then tend to consume too much meat, and the meat is often from questionable sources. Also, the kinds of meats (bacon, pork, etc.) consumed can contain nitrates that have been shown to be harmful to a baby.

As a soon-to-be new mom, you must be careful about keeping the right balance to ensure you get all the nutrients needed for your growing baby. Again, as with vegan and veggie moms, Paleo moms do not consume enough deep-pigmented veggies. A high protein diet can also be very taxing to the kidneys, and therefore can cause challenges with digestion and constipation.

Personally, I am a pagan, or you might say I follow a plant-based paleo diet (if we have to put a label on our foods). This type of diet works best for me; it makes me feel balanced. It consists of lots of veggies and greens, nuts and seeds, healthy fats, some low-glycemic fruits like berries and pears, and lean proteins, mostly from wild fish and fowl. If you are interested, there is a simple plant-based paleo diet outline in the back of the book. Remember, this book is about finding your balance and what is right for you.

HOW MUCH WEIGHT GAIN IS HEALTHY

Here's what the guidelines for BMI (basal metabolic index) suggest if you fall into what is considered the normal range. That range is between 18 and 25. If you are in this range, then the average and healthy weight gain is between twenty to thirty pounds with twenty-five pounds being the average. That being said, it is a myth that you need to eat for two. You probably don't need much more extra calories until you reach the third trimester. What counts is the quality of the calories you consume, not the quantity.

If your BMI is less than 18, you should gain some healthy weight. If your BMI is 25–30 or higher, then you are overweight and, therefore, you should gain less weight to avoid pregnancy problems down the road. If you are overweight and want to get pregnant, I strongly suggest you seek support before conception. It will be much better for you and much better for baby.

KEEPING MY IMMUNE SYSTEM STRONG

The best way to keep your immune system strong for a balanced and beautiful pregnancy is to eat well, exercise, and keep stress to a minimum:

- Avoid simple sugars and simple carbs.
- Enjoy lots of greens.
- Get adequate calcium, magnesium, and vitamin D3.
- Take a good probiotic.
- Download the app called "Headspace" and meditate

Gut health is critical for managing immune health. Enjoy your pregnancy and celebrate all the things you do each day to nurture yourself and your baby. If this is your first pregnancy, try to stay balanced and not stress about every detail. Stress has a huge impact on the immune system and therefore a significant impact on the health of your baby.

Stay grounded and stay in the moment. Love yourself and love your child.

I AM SO TIRED. HANDLING FATIGUE.

Your body is going through a lot of significant changes at a relatively rapid pace, so you are going to need additional nutrients to support these changes.

First: Make sure you are getting adequate sleep. The body repairs itself during sleep, and this is when the liver does most of its work to rid the body of toxins.

Second: Dehydration could be the cause of your fatigue. Make sure you are getting plenty of fresh water, at a minimum 80 oz. Per day. As discussed, you will need even more in the third trimester.

Third: Toxins could also be a likely culprit. If you are eating poorly and mismanaging your blood sugar, you will feel tired.

If you are getting good sleep, eating well, are well-hydrated and still feel fatigued, you should check in with your physician to make sure you do not have a hidden infection or are low in a particular nutrient.

Your fatigue could also mean you need more nutrients, especially folate, B12, vitamin D, and B-complex. (A special note about iron: Unless your blood work shows a deficiency, we suggest eating foods rich in iron. Supplemental iron can cause digestive stress and's hard to absorb.

You should also make sure your prenatal vitamin is high quality. You can self-test the quality of your prenatal supplements by dropping them into white vinegar heated to ninety-nine degrees. If they dissolve in thirty minutes or less, then your body will absorb them. If they do not dissolve completely, then you have just learned that you have an expensive pee and it is time to upgrade your prenatal vitamin.

CHAPTER 4: THE SECOND TRIMESTER

STAYING THE COURSE WITH GOOD NUTRITION

For most women, the second trimester is the period when they feel good, and some moms even feel great. You have a baby bump, your hormones seem in balance, your nausea it has subsided, and your energy level is back to normal.

If you had some struggles during your first trimester, trying to eat all the nutritious foods we talked about in chapter one and two, then this is the time to make a better effort. It is never too late to do this, and better late than never. Don't beat yourself up about the past; just start now and look forward and stay grounded in the present moment.

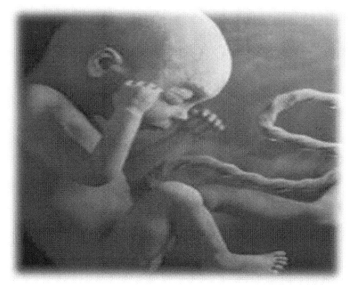

It is also the time that you should have more energy, so it is time to get back on track with a regular exercise routine or sign up for a prenatal yoga class in your area. (This is also an excellent way to meet other pregnant moms.)

BABY'S BONES ARE DEVELOPING: WHY YOU NEED MAGNESIUM, CALCIUM, AND ANTIOXIDANTS

The second trimester is the time when your baby is developing skin and bones. It is a period when there is rapid growth and a need for the minerals that build strong, healthy bones. We talked a bit about the many benefits of magnesium. Remember that magnesium also works in conjunction with calcium and phosphorus to build bones.

If you are following a healthy eating plan and you are filling in with whole food supplements, you should be getting enough of these essential bone-building nutrients.

It is a time when collagen is also important. We talked a bit about collagen, so you already know it is a key building block for many of your baby's structural tissues like cartilage, tendons, and ligaments, as well as healthy skin, nails, and hair. One of the central building blocks for collagen is vitamin C. Fortunately, vitamin C is found in a lot of foods. Adding a squeeze of lime or lemon to your drinking water is an easy and safe way to make sure you are getting vitamin C in a natural form.

RAMPING UP THE CALORIES A LITTLE

I am a little reluctant to suggest this, as most moms will take me at my word and perhaps over-indulge. You will need to up the calories a bit to accommodate this growth spurt.

We suggest making sure you are eating adequate protein and healthy fats. These are the two areas to focus on to ensure you are getting enough of the right kind of calories. Refer to our protein guide in the back of the book for more information.

The other thing to mention here is that you are not eating for two. It is key to listen to your body really. If you are in tune and connected with your body, you will know what you need.

WHY ALL CALORIES ARE NOT CREATED EQUAL

The quality of the food you eat is paramount. The term "calorie" is used a lot, and it is a measure of energy we still see used in conjunction with weight loss programs and the like. For example, if you gained one pound or lost one pound without changing anything, you would have added or taken away 3,500 calories, respectively.

That being said, you want to consume food that is nutrient dense so that you obtain the maximum benefits for your unborn baby and yourself. The other interesting thing is when you eat nutrient-dense food, you feel more satisfied and energized. When you eat empty calories, your body does not get the nutrients it needs, and you therefore feel hungry.

STAYING HYDRATED: WATER, WATER, AND MORE WATER

Staying hydrated during pregnancy is very important. As discussed earlier, water is a fundamental building block for a healthy baby, and it is especially important during the formation of the amniotic fluid early in the first trimester.

Again, if you are drinking plenty of water and it seems to be going right for you, add a pinch of sea salt or Himalayan salt (for electrolytes) to your water. You might also need other additional electrolytes, and if so please talk to your health practitioner about what is best for you.

We also suggest that you don't drink water out of plastic bottles; make sure the water is filtered; it is best consumed at room temperature.

Some of the negative symptoms associated with pregnancy such as muscle cramps, headaches, constipation, fatigue, etc., are often signs of dehydration that can be easily cured by drinking enough clean filtered water. If you hate drinking water, add some lemon, cucumber, or pineapple to give it a little flavor.

CHAPTER 5: THIRD TRIMESTER- PREPARING FOR BIRTH

The third trimester is a time when your unborn child has completed the development of their primary structures with some fine-tuning yet to be done. It is the time when your baby grows rapidly and prepares to live and thrive outside the womb.

All of a sudden it will seem like you are carrying this huge ball in front of your body that you need to accommodate. Your center of gravity changes and the extra weight along with the modification in your silhouette can cause a stiff back and pelvic pain.

Keeping up with your prenatal yoga, the exercise of your choice and healthy food choices is as important as ever. The added stress of the weight gain and additional fluid volume can take a toll on your body.

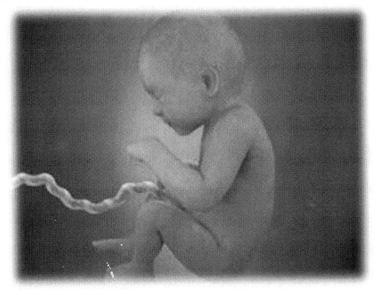

If you have not done so already, you might want to consider adding prenatal chiropractic care, acupuncture, or prenatal massage to your pregnancy care plan.

It is also a time of great joy as you prepare to celebrate with friends and family by planning a baby shower or a ceremonial blessing. It is also a time to finalize the plan you and your partner would like for the birth of your beautiful baby.

Hypno Birthing teaches you how to go into the moment of calm during the birth process, which has enormous benefits. That peaceful place of reducing stress and allows the body to stimulate oxytocin. Oxytocin is the hormone that allows "relaxing" to do its work on the muscles and ligaments for an easier birth process.

AVOIDING LATE PREGNANCY PROBLEMS

We hope you have been eating a clean, healthy diet, exercising regularly, and keeping stress to a minimum and, therefore, do not have any late pregnancy problems. However, if you do, we want to provide you with some suggestions and support.

Also, it is important to know that the risks from gestational diabetes do not end at delivery. What you decide to do postpartum is also super important. Often this is an area that is not discussed, and it is one of the most important aspects of your blood sugar handling plan, as it affects your and your baby's future health.

WHAT HAPPENS NEXT IF I FAIL THE TEST?

Not all moms who take the glucose challenge test are overweight. Some are following a paleo or low carb diet and therefore the sugary drink given at the glucose challenge test will cause a spike in blood sugar levels the body is not used to.

There are also moms out there who are not doing a good job of managing their blood glucose on a day-to-day basis. Those moms are often hypoglycemic (have low blood sugar) or follow a vegetarian or vegan diet (too many carbs and not enough protein and veggies). Then, some moms who have had hormonal issues in the past or are currently under high stress, also fail the test.

It is a perfect time to learn about your unique makeup and what foods, drinks, stressors, etc., affect your blood sugar levels. In some folks, a seemingly benign type of food can cause an increase in glucose levels. Examples I have seen are chicken, salmon, oranges, tomatoes, peanuts, and rice.

If you failed the glucose challenge test, this is like the check engine light coming on telling you, "Hey, you need to make changes." Everyone has a unique profile, and this is where we can help understand your triggers.

GETTING BLOOD GLUCOSE UNDER CONTROL

First, if you are eating and drinking sugar and sweets, it is time to stop. Increase your intake of whole foods, VEGGIES in particular, and make sure you are getting adequate amounts of protein and healthy fats.

Second, get a glucose monitor and some glucose strips so you can control your blood glucose levels.

DEALING WITH HEARTBURN

Heartburn is caused by the contents of the stomach backing up via the esophageal sphincter. The primary cause of this problem is that you are not digesting your food well. Therefore, it is putrefying in the stomach and irritating the sphincter. The sphincter can be aggravated by certain foods, the extra pressure of the growing belly, a lack of stomach acid, or additional stress.

Under stress, the body is in sympathetic mode, which means all the blood from the central organs goes to the extremities, and hydrochloric acid production in the stomach shuts down. What you want to do is make sure that after you eat, take a few minutes to relax and breathe. Optimal digestion occurs when the body is in parasympathetic mode. That is why it is often called "rest and digest."

It is also helpful to speak with your healthcare practitioner to see if adding some digestive enzymes or HCL (hydrochloric acid) support will help relieve your symptoms. You could also take a two-ounce shot of apple cider vinegar before each meal to stimulate stomach acid production.

We do not recommend the use of antacids and proton pump inhibitors like Pepcid because they make the overall problem worse and can cause other issues down the road. They treat the symptoms and not the cause, which, as discussed, is usually NOT enough stomach acid.

It could also be that you need to add more calcium to your diet. Calcium and HCL work together in the stomach to provide the optimal pH for digestion and maintaining a healthy immune system. (Bacteria, viruses, and pathogens like E. coli, etc., cannot live in an acidic environment, so optimal pH in the stomach is important for overall health.)

Enjoying smaller meals more often could also be beneficial as well as avoiding possible triggers such as spicy foods or foods made with harmful fats.

The higher your BMI (body mass index), the greater the possibility of heartburn. If you suspect you have a stomach ulcer, take action and visit your healthcare practitioner to discuss natural solutions.

HOW TO AVOID CONSTIPATION?

Constipation is uncomfortable; not only that but if one of your primary elimination processes is not working well, it means toxins stay inside your body for too long. This can cause immune problems.

There are some things that could be the cause of your constipation challenges. It could be the lack of fiber in your diet, so make sure you are getting enough—yet another great reason to increase the intake of veggies and greens. If you have not already done so, add our Ultimate Protein Smoothie to your diet and be sure to add the suggested fiber options.

You could be dehydrated. As discussed in earlier chapters, pregnant moms need lots of water.

It could be due to a lack of exercise. Exercise keeps all the fluids in the body moving well and also massages the internal organs of the digestive tract.

It could be that you are not digesting your foods well, and therefore they are not broken down and absorbed. These undigested foods enter the digestive tract like a log and have a hard time passing through.

Digestive enzyme support could be helpful along with additional HCL (hydrochloric acid).

Some iron supplements can cause constipation, and for this reason, we recommend food sources of iron like almonds, kelp, spinach, and grass-fed meats to help keep iron levels up. Iron also needs vitamin C to be absorbed well. If you do need to supplement iron, then we like a liquid formula called Floradix. For additional vitamin C, add lemon or lime to your water.

You could be having thyroid problems. The thyroid controls the function of your basal metabolic rate. If the thyroid is "hypo" your basal metabolic rate will be slow and therefore so will the rate of digestion, absorption, and elimination.

Pregnancy is a time when hormones can fluctuate a lot. The endocrine glands like the thyroid are all linked together via a positive and negative feedback system, so when one gland is hyper (too fast) or hypo it can affect the others. If you suspect you are having issues with your thyroid, please check with your healthcare provider ASAP. The most common cause of miscarriage is linked to thyroid fluctuations.

It is also possible that you might have an imbalance in your gut flora. Taking a good probiotic at night before bed will help rebalance the gut.

If you have addressed all of the above and you are still having problems, add a magnesium supplement to the probiotic at night.

THE BEST WAY TO THINK ABOUT STRESS AND YOUR UNBORN CHILD

Some anxious moms feel good in their third trimester. They say they've never felt better. Why is that? The answer is that mom is taking adrenal support from her baby. What happens next is that baby's adrenal glands are depleted, and more often than the not baby tends to be sensitive, have sleep issues, or be anxious, fussy, suffer from ADHD, and the like. We see this a lot in children who were the first born in their family, and particularly if they were the first born after a previous miscarriage.

We are learning more and more that the womb is not a sterile environment and that mom's environment (mind, body, and spirit) has a direct effect on the environment of a baby in the womb.

Keeping stress low during pregnancy will be beneficial for mom and baby. It is where dad can play a significant role along with other members of their support team. Getting out and in touch with nature or deep breathing exercises are also great stress relievers. For me, I enjoy yoga, a walk along the beach, planting a garden, and dinner with good friends. These are all good stress relievers for me.

I strongly suggest you find what works for you and practice it often throughout your pregnancy and your life.

CHAPTER 6: THE FOURTH TRIMESTER: CONGRATULATIONS! YOU HAVE A NEW BABY!

I have been lucky enough to be in the room after birth on several occasions. The energy, wonder, and love that flows between mom, dad, and their new baby are like nothing else I have ever experienced. It is like being in a dreamland, and something powerful has just taken place and, in fact, it has! You are holding a human who has a piece of your genic blueprint and that of your partner.

I sincerely hope you had a gentle and beautiful birth. I hope it was what you wanted for yourself and your child. If not, then that is OK, and it is time to move forward with the healing process. Birth is exhilarating and stressful at the same time. It takes a lot of energy, so hopefully, you have taken some time to cocoon as a family.

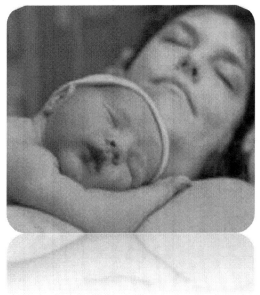

If you have been following along with us, then you have healthy practices in place, and your resilience factor should be high and the healing process much quicker.

Having some things in place before birth can be helpful. Making sure you have some healthy foods stocked away in the freezer, engaging the help of a food service, or a hiring postpartum doula are some of the things we suggest. It will allow you the time you all need to rest and recoup and settle into a sleep, wake, and feeding routine with your new baby.

BOUNCING BACK AFTER BIRTH

It is normal to feel a little of the baby blues after giving birth. During pregnancy, your placenta has guided your endocrine system to increase progesterone levels to a higher level than you might have experienced before. Some moms tell me they only feel great when they are pregnant. Progesterone is the feel-good, calming hormone; and once you have given birth and the placenta has been removed, your hormone level of progesterone drops. This abrupt drop can take a little adjustment.

Some women choose to have their placentas encapsulated. It is a process where the placenta is removed and dried and put into capsule form. The idea is that you take these tablets postpartum. This process has been shown to help moms combat the baby blues.

For more information, we suggest you talk to your doula, midwife, or health care provider. Do your research to ensure that this is the right decision for you.

If you had a caesarean birth, we suggest you treat this as a recovery from major surgery. You will need to detox the drugs and antibiotics and support tissue healing. To do that, we suggest adding a proteolytic enzyme to your diet to support tissue healing. These enzymes taken away from food will help significantly with recovery and act as an anti-inflammatory.

Continue with your probiotics to support healthy gut flora following a course of antibiotics, and in some cases, you might need to increase your dose for a short time.

Make sure you drink plenty of clean water, not only to flush out toxins and tissue damage but also to encourage adequate milk supply. In some cases, you will want to increase your antioxidants like vitamin C for a short period to support healing.

Consider Arnica, a homeopathic remedy to help with internal bruising and trauma.

Lastly, continue to eat well to support the healing process and to provide your baby with healthy breast milk.

FOODS THAT SUPPORT LACTATION AND MILK PRODUCTION

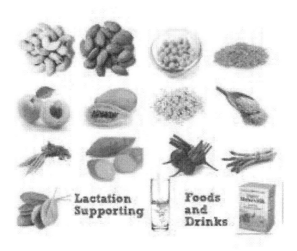

Research shows us that breastfeeding is the very best option for a new baby. Study after study concludes that breastfed babies thrive and outperform on cognitive skill tests versus those who were bottle-fed.

Nature innately knows how to formulate the right nutrients your child needs. We are aware that in today's world it is challenging to breastfeed your baby until they are naturally weaned. However, we are firmly suggesting you allow three months as the minimum time frame. The longer you can breastfeed, the better for your baby. We should also mention that the bonding that occurs between mom and baby during breastfeeding and the act of providing nourishment from one human to another can't be described as anything other than very special.

Breast milk contains mother's colostrum, which is very high in antibodies. That along with a vaginal birth provides a jump-start to a healthy immune system for your new baby. Breast milk is also easier for your baby to digest than most standard baby formulas, unless, of course, you, mom, are eating foods that cause you or baby to have a histamine (allergic) response. Histamine is high when you are exposed to something the body sees as a pathogen. It triggers the inflammation cascade.

Typically, I have found that if moms eat a lot of processed foods like dairy or foods with soy, newborns can have digestive challenges trying to break down these proteins.

The symptoms that show up in your child are typically gas, bloating, digestive pain, and increased spit-ups, etc. In some cases, we have added digestive support for mom so she can break down the proteins and therefore baby's digestive problems are resolved. If not, then it is best to do an elimination diet and avoid all dairy and soy to see if the problem resolves itself.

HOW DOES DIET AFFECT BREAST MILK?

Your diet has an impact on your breast milk. Breast milk can taste and smell different at each feeding based on what you have consumed. Your baby is being exposed to all the different flavors you eat and drink through your breast milk. Baby will particularly notice if you had a spicy meal, as they will be consuming the spice too.

If you experience challenges with breastfeeding, we recommend you contact a lactation consultant. They are experts and will be able to provide information and resources to help support you through this new experience.

We have talked about all the benefits of breastfeeding; however, in some cases, breastfeeding is not possible, so we suggest you don't stress and look for milk formula options that do not contain SOY.

We like a recipe derived from the Weston Price Foundation. Dave Asprey, who is a published nutrition expert and author of the Better Baby Book, also recommends this method.

Formula Recipe:

- 1 cup of milk-based powdered formula
- 29 oz. of filtered water
- One large raw organic egg yolk
- ½ teaspoon of cod liver oil
- Raw organic cream
- One teaspoon of pure oil (sunflower, walnut, sesame [rotate oils])
- One teaspoon of MCT (medium-cha triglyceride) oil

1. Blend thoroughly and refrigerate. When heating put the bottle in hot water and do not overheat, as the formula will denature.

2. There are goat milk based recipes available if your baby does not tolerate whey.

TAKING PROBIOTICS WHILE I AM BREASTFEEDING

Yes, you can. Taking probiotics is of particular importance if you had a caesarean birth or IV antibiotics due to GBS (group B strep). In some cases, we suggest a probiotic for baby in addition to one for mom. In this case, it is typically when the birth has been difficult, and there has been the need for surgery or additional antibiotic medication.

We have also suggested additional probiotics for babies who have come to us having experienced immune challenges and are having difficulty with feeding and absorbing nutrients.

There are some great baby probiotic formulas out there; however, we like to use mom's probiotic. Only break open the capsule and put a little bit on your finger and have the baby suck it off your finger. That way baby can absorb the probiotic quickly. It can begin to work and does not taste bad.

CONTINUING PRENATAL VITAMINS

We suggest you continue to eat well, consuming a variety of whole, nutritious foods, and continue to take your prenatal supplements for at least three months and then switch over to my

Fab Five.

The Fab Five is well rounded and covers a lot of health and wellness bases. Together with a proper diet, they can keep you healthy. At a minimum, we recommend taking the following supplements every day: probiotic, fish oil, a B-complex, a mineral supplement, and a digestive enzyme. Here's why:

1. Probiotics

Probiotics support healthy gut flora, maintain a healthy gut environment, and improve nutrient digestion and absorption. They support GI immune health and are an excellent **adjunct to antibiotic** therapy, which has been overprescribed for years. Probiotics are best taken at night, as this is when your digestive system does its work.

2. Omega-3 Fatty Acids

Omega-3s are an excellent source of DHA and EPA essential fatty acids. These are called the GOOD Fats. Omega-3s act as an anti-inflammatory and support optimal cardiovascular function help keep blood stable and support brain health.

3. A B Vitamin Complex

B-complex vitamins contribute to improving nerve conductivity, support blood sugar imbalances, and help with hypotension (low blood pressure) and drug and alcohol use. A lack of Vitamin B can lead to depression and anxiety. It is a must-have if you are a vegan or vegetarian because you are not getting the most bioavailable for the body B vitamins from your diet.

4. A Mineral Supplement

For most of us, the best mineral supplement comes in the form of a calcium-magnesium-vitamin D3 combo. In some cases, zinc is the mineral that would be most beneficial.

5. Digestive Enzymes

For most of us, digestive enzymes are a combo of pepsin and hydrochloric acid (HCL). Stress reduces the production of HCL, and therefore we often suffer from digestive issues due to the body's inability to break down food.

Digestive enzymes help with indigestion, gas, and bloating. They also help with calcium, anemia, and iron absorption. If you have sharp breath, they are a must.

Other than the Fab Five there is a possibility that you might need to increase your consumption of antioxidants like vitamin C, vitamin E, and vitamin A.

The necessity of iron decreases after birth, so we suggest you stop supplementing with iron and instead eat iron-rich foods. However, if you had a lot of blood loss during birth, you should talk with your physician about having your iron levels checked.

If you have questions, it is always prudent to check in with your health and wellness doctor for your unique needs.

POSTPARTUM WEIGHT LOSS

If this were your first pregnancy, you would no doubt expect that once you had your baby your belly bump would magically disappear. The truth is, it can take a little while for the uterus and the increase in fluid volume during pregnancy to get back to normal.

The combination of the weight of the baby, the placenta, amniotic fluid, and water and blood loss add up to about twelve plus pounds. If you have been following along with our plan, you would have gained no more than twenty-five pounds. The way to look at this is that you have lost half your baby weight very quickly even though you still feel swollen and pregnant the first day or two after delivery.

The days following birth can be hectic as you, your family, and your baby establish the patterns for sleeping, eating, and living. I always suggest that parents take time during the first week to ten days to cocoon and develop rhythms that work for everyone in the household. There is a ton of information out there about how many feedings babies should be having, how much sleep, how much poop, how much weight the baby should be gaining, etc.

Having a baby is not like having a wearable device like a Fitbit with beepers going off telling you when to do this and when to do that. Can they be helpful? Yes. However, building a human is an organic process that requires careful attention.

I must admit I am a little shocked at how big the electronic baby changer pad has been. I am not sure I would expose my newborn child to the effects of EMF so I could monitor their every oz., poop, heart rate, etc. when there is still so much unknown about the effects.

Once you and your family have established a routine that is best for all, it is time to get back on the exercise bandwagon. Start with walking, which you and baby can do together, and then gradually increase the intensity and amount. If you had a caesarean birth or other complications during birth, then it will take longer to recover and get back to a regular exercise routine. There are some excellent resources available for you like FIT4MOM.com or post-natal mom and baby yoga classes.

It is not the time to put weight loss and possible dietary restrictions above nutrient-dense foods. When you balance your energy with the right amount of exercise and foods for you, you will never have to worry about weight gain. This rule applies whether you are pregnant or not.

WHY IS IT IMPORTANT TO TAKE CARE OF YOURSELF FIRST THEN BABY?

This is the area where the wheels fall off for most new parents. They do a good job of staying fit and relatively healthy before having a family. Then the first baby comes along, and they are now consumed 24/7 with the needs of the child and they neglect the healthy behaviors they once had in place.

Stress levels go up, sleep is almost always challenging, and slowly but surely that can lead to less-than-optimal diet choices. Even the most grounded, well-informed moms and dads worry and stress over every detail in the first few weeks of their newborn's life. It is a natural instinct to nurture. However, if you find yourself over-obsessing and neglecting yourself, then take a step back and inhale some deep breaths and trust that all will be OK. Ask yourself what advice you would give to someone else.

What you don't want is to fast-forward a few years, and the kids are now off to school, and you find yourself 10/20/30 pounds overweight and feeling bad. What happened? Where did the time go? The best thing for you and your family long-term is to make a chance to take care of yourself. Kids want parents who are full of vitality and energy. They need good role models so they, too, can grow up to be healthy and vital adults. I can't stress this enough.

DRINKING ALCOHOL WHILE BREASTFEEDING

The decision is yours. Research shows that drinking alcohol can inhibit lactation and in turn reduce your milk supply. If you are having challenges with milk production, then abstinence is the best course of action.

If you choose to drink, then do so right after a feeding, so your body has a chance to metabolize the alcohol. If you know you are going out to have a couple of drinks with friends, we suggest you plan and pump extra milk before consuming alcohol.

A note: The liver will detox alcohol first. So, know that if you drink, your major organ of detoxification will be busy dealing with the alcohol.

CHAPTER 7: HIGH-RISK PREGNANCY

A high-risk pregnancy is when a condition puts the mother, baby or both at an increased risk. You are more likely to have a high-risk pregnancy if you:

- Are overweight (especially if it is by more than 22kg)
- Smoke
- Have seizures
- Have diabetes
- Use drugs or alcohol
- Are younger than 18 or older than 35

- Have a history of genetic defects or
- You are having twins/triplets, etc.

Just because you have these factors does not automatically mean you have a high-risk pregnancy; and the opposite is true, just because you have no pre-existing health issues will not guarantee a healthy pregnancy. You are also at more risk if you have had any of the above issues/complications in a previous pregnancy.

If you have a pre-existing condition, you need to discuss the pros and cons of pregnancy with your GP and supervising consultant. There are many variables to consider and you need an expert to advise you

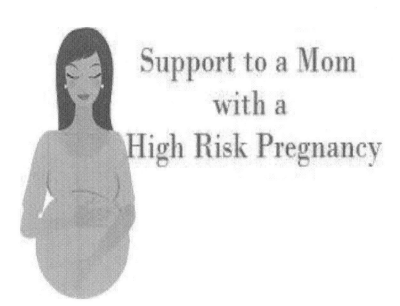

HYPEREMESIS GRAVIDARUM (HG):

This condition affects about 1% of pregnant women and is an extreme form of nausea and vomiting. It is not known why some women get it, and others don't, but some evidence shows it runs in families; and if you experienced HG in a previous pregnancy, you are more likely to get it in subsequent ones. Some tips to help alleviate symptoms are:

- Rest
- Staying hydrated
- Avoiding nausea triggers
- Emotional and physical support

Not all tips work for all women, and it can be a case of trial and error to find the ones that work for you. Be that as it may, some medications can help, including in the early stages of pregnancy, e.g. anti-sickness drugs, steroids, and vitamins B6 & B12.

N.B.: If you are unable to keep down food and fluids, contact your doctor, as you can become dehydrated very quickly when suffering from HG; and you may need to be admitted to hospital for intravenous fluid therapy.

GESTATIONAL DIABETES:

It is caused because the placenta produces hormones that lead to an increase of sugar in your blood. Your pancreas usually produces enough insulin to control this. If not, then it will cause your blood sugar to rise, and you will develop gestational diabetes. Symptoms may not necessarily arise but can include: feeling tired; being very thirsty; weeing a lot; a dry mouth, and infections like thrush, or blurred vision. Please make an appointment to see your health professional so that you can be monitored more closely. Gestational diabetes may mean you go into premature labor, so your baby will be monitored to make sure they do not show any signs of distress. After birth, your baby may need to have blood tests regularly, as they may have low-blood sugar, while they adapt to making the right amount of insulin.

PREECLAMPSIA:

It affects some women, usually in the second half of pregnancy, and it can even happen after their baby is born. When you see your midwife, they will monitor your blood pressure and test a urine sample. Preeclampsia is one of the things they are checking for. Early signs are high blood pressure and protein found in your urine. Other symptoms include excess swelling of the hands, feet, and legs; severe headaches; and vision issues. If you notice any of these symptoms, you need to seek the advice of your midwife or GP immediately. In most cases, preeclampsia does not cause any problems, and it improves after delivery.

N.B.: There is a risk that preeclampsia can become 'eclampsia.' These are seizures, that can put both the mother and baby at risk. Contact your GP if you have any concerns.

ECTOPIC PREGNANCY:

An ectopic pregnancy can occur when the fertilized egg implants outside of the uterus, usually in the fallopian tube. Symptoms to look out for are:

- A missed period (some women may not know they are pregnant)
- Vaginal bleeding
- Pain in your lower abdomen – on one side
- Pain in the tip of your shoulder (no one is sure why this occurs)
- Discomfort is weeing or peeing

An ectopic pregnancy may grow large enough that it causes a fallopian tube to rupture. It is an emergency, and you need surgery to repair or remove the fallopian tube. Signs of a fracture are: feeling very dizzy or faint; nausea or vomiting; looking very pale; or a sharp, sudden, acute pain in your tummy. Seek medical help immediately.

PLACENTA PREVIA:

It is where the placenta lies unusually low in the uterus, and it may be near or over the surface of the cervix. Early in pregnancy, it does not cause a problem; but later it can be an issue, as it will block your baby's way out. They will record the position of your placenta when you have your second scan; and if you are found to have placenta previa, they will perform another scan at around the 32-week mark. If the placenta is low, it puts you at higher risk of bleeding throughout your pregnancy and labor, and this bleeding may be heavy, which puts you and your baby at risk. Your consultant may recommend that you are admitted to hospital towards the end of your pregnancy so that they can monitor you closely, and emergency treatment is at hand. They will recommend you have a caesarian if the placenta is completely blocking your cervix.

N.B.: If you experience bright red (painless) bleeding during the last few months of pregnancy, contact your midwife or doctor immediately.

PLACENTAL ABRUPTION:

If a placental tear occurs, you may notice vaginal bleeding and should seek medical attention. However, approximately 90% of these tears can heal themselves, but they may also put you at an increased risk of a miscarriage, premature labor or placental abruption. It is a complication of pregnancy that means the placenta has separated from the wall of the uterus. It can deprive your baby of oxygen and nutrients but also cause severe bleeding that could be dangerous to you both.

N.B.: if you notice any of the following: vaginal bleeding, abdominal pain, rapid contractions, or your 'baby bump' is tender seek medical attention immediately.

PREMATURE LABOR:

Early labor can be divided into groups:

- Extremely early: under 28 weeks gestation
- Very early: 28 to 32 weeks
- Late prematurity: 32 to 37 weeks

Although it is important a baby gets as close to the due date as possible, sometimes things happen that are outside your control. Some factors mean you may be more at risk of premature labor. These are:

- Multiple pregnancies
- Lifestyle factors (smoking, recreational drugs, high caffeine intake; poor diet/being underweight)
- Maternal age (under 20, over 35)

- Infections (chlamydia, untreated bladder infection)
- Cervical incompetence (the cervix opens too soon, and labor follows)

While some of these cannot be avoided, others can. It is important to receive proper antenatal care, have regular checkups and maintain a healthy lifestyle. If you are concerned, contact your GP/midwife immediately.

SOCIAL FACTORS

Older mums

You may hear the term elderly primigravida. It is from the age of 35, so not that old really, but pregnancy from this age may come with additional risks.

Most older mom's these days have chosen to delay pregnancy. Although some women have medical reasons, e.g. repeated miscarriages, fertility issues. Much more elderly mums have decided to delay pregnancy for social/personal reasons, and they tend to be better educated, more confident and financially stable. You do however need to be aware of associated risks, some of which are:

- Decreased fertility
- Chromosomal abnormalities

- Developing high blood pressure or diabetes
- Multiple births
- Birth intervention (labor induction, forceps)
- Caesarean section

N.B: It is best to talk to your doctor before trying to conceive. They can give you a thorough checkup and advice to ensure you are in good general health and refer you to a specialist if you have any specific issues that need addressing.

TEEN PREGNANCY

Most girls usually start their periods about the age of 12, and teen pregnancy is defined as occurring between the age of 13 and 19 years. Teens (both girls and boys) need to be educated to realize that girls can become pregnant as soon as they begin to ovulate, so they need to practice safe sex if they are to avoid becoming pregnant. If you are a teenager, pregnant and reading this, please talk to an adult you trust: mum or dad, a school counselor/teacher, or call a support helpline. Above all, you need to get help/advice and medical support for you and your baby, whether you choose to continue with the pregnancy or not.

BED REST

Some pregnant women are advised to stay on bed rest (for a short or extended period). They may be at risk of complications such as high blood pressure, pre-eclampsia; vaginal bleeding (placenta previa, placental abruption), premature labor, threatened miscarriage, cervical insufficiency, or there may be growth issues with the baby. Some women may need to reduce their activity, or reduce their stress levels, and being put on bed rest is a way to reduce unnecessary physical activities. However, being put on bed rest is not without its issues. You may be more likely to experience heartburn, constipation, or you may just feel down since your lifestyle is curtailed.

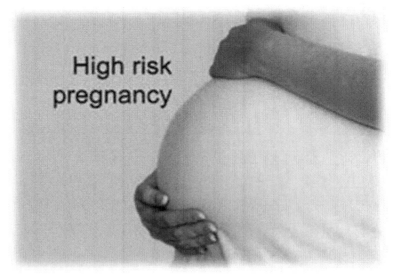

CHAPTER 8: WHAT DO I NEED TO TAKE INTO HOSPITAL

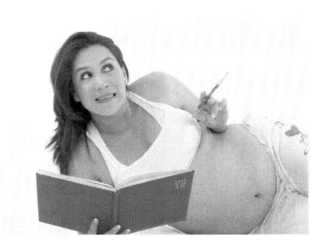

What goes in a hospital bag and when should I get it ready? Regardless of whether you are having a home, hospital or midwifery-unit birth, you need to pack a bag, so everything is in one place and case of emergencies at least two weeks before your due date. Your midwife will provide you with a list tailored to your particular hospital/midwifery unit, but here are some things that you might want to include:

- Your birth plan, if you have written one.
- Medications/list of drugs for any pre-existing conditions/illnesses you may have.
- Things to help you relax, or pass the time (music, magazines).
- Loose and comfy clothing to wear during labor. Natural fibers are a better choice than human-made, as they let your body breathe more. You will probably need a few changes throughout labor, so make sure to pack about three sets. Some women may prefer to be naked throughout labor, but it is probably wise to pack them just in case. Don't forget to pack a comfortable outfit to wear home!
- About 24 extra-absorbent sanitary pads (maternity ones with wings are a good idea).
- Sponge/cloth or a water-spray to help keep you calm during labor.
- Front-opening, or loose-fitting nightie or tops for breastfeeding; 2 or 3 supportive but comfortable bras (make sure to take nursing bras if you are breastfeeding).
- Breast pads.

- At least 5 or 6 pairs of pants.
- Toiletry bag;
- Towels.
- Dressing gown and slippers
- Clothing (make sure you include a hat) and nappies (diapers) for the baby.
- A shawl to wrap the baby in.
- A camera to capture those all-important first moments.

Think about getting to and from the hospital and make sure you have a contingency plan in the case of unexpected problems with transport. Reflect on the route you will take, allow for unforeseen hold-ups, e.g. roadworks. Remember, you can always call an ambulance!

N.B.: make sure you have a rear-facing car seat (and you disable any associated airbags). Please get expert advice, and ensure you are aware of the new car seat regulations, which came into effect in March of 2017.

If you plan to have a home birth, you will need to discuss this with your midwife to ensure you have everything required. But at the very least, you will need clean linen and towels available for the attendant to use, sanitary pads and clothing for when your baby arrives. You also need to think about where in the home you want to give birth and if you need to hire specialist equipment, e.g. a birthing pool.

Many people have mobile phones, but it can be handy to keep a written list of important contact details: your hospital and midwife phone numbers, your partner/birth partner's phone number, your hospital reference number, as they will ask for this when you phone to say you are on your way.

HOME EQUIPMENT CONSIDERATIONS

Babies require a lot of attention and come with a lot of baggage! You may be thinking where do I start, as there are many items to buy before your baby is born. If this is your first baby, you may want to buy everything in sight, but just be aware you may find that you don't need it all straight away. You will find family and friends will want to help let them!

Below is a list of items you may need immediately:

- Moses basket and stand
- Sheets and waffle blanket
- Changing table
- Baby monitor
- Baby bouncer
- Pram

- Breast feeding pillow (if required)
- Sterilizer and bottles
- Baby formula (if bottle feeding)
- Baby bath
- Nappy bag
- Scented nappy sacks

Possible purchases are:

- Bottle warmer (a jug of hot water will suffice)
- Breast pump
- Nappy bucket (for terry nappies to be collected by an agency)
- Nappy disposal Bin (these are specialist bins that lock odors away!)
- Dummies (if you think you want your baby to have one)

These things can wait to be purchased later:

- Cot
- High chair
- Safety gate and catches
- Buggy

Newborns need a lot of attention. Make sure you gather a supply of necessary equipment a couple of weeks before your due date.

Some of the visible items your baby will need are:

- Nappies (terry or disposable);
- Baby wipes
- Baby powder
- Nappy rash ointment/cream
- Baby oil/lotion
- Baby shampoo

Less obvious items are:

- Nail scissors (specifically for newborns)
- Baby brush
- Baby thermometer
- Laundry powder that is hypoallergenic
- Thermometer for your bathtub (many parents use the elbow in the water technique, satisfactorily), but whatever you use, be sure to put the cold water into the bath first then the hot. This way you avoid the possible risk of burns to the baby

During the first weeks after your baby's arrival you may not leave the house often to buy all the necessary items, so make sure you accept help when offered. Children go through tons of nappies but do not overstock, as they change size frequently. If you chose not to breastfeed or cannot, you would need to buy formula milk.

N.B.: Do not makeup bottles with water straight from the tap. It needs to be freshly boiled and left to cool, for no more than 30 minutes before you make up the milk.

You are going to want to buy clothes for your baby, but please remember many people may gift you baby clothes. An item you ought to buy is a swaddle blanket; this keeps your child warm and comfortable after they are born.

OTHER ITEMS TO BUY INCLUDE:

- Baby-grows/onesies
- Socks
- No-scratch mittens
- Leggings
- T-shirts
- Cardigans/jumpers
- Coats
- Hats
- Bibs
- Burp cloths/muslins

Bear in mind that depending on when your child is born, weather plays a factor when deciding which clothes to buy. Babies grow fast, so there is no need to buy too many clothes before they are born. It's not just your child that needs things ready at home for; after the birth, you will too. Some items are nursing bras, breast pads, sanitary pads, nipple cream, comfy clothing, a supply of nutritious snacks and foods.

CHAPTER 9: TAKING CARE OF HER

Your BMP must go through a lot of changes. Her hard-won figure will soon be transformed. Her mobility will decrease. She may experience constant nausea. She's suffering all of this in the name of having a baby with you. So, your best possible move is to attempt to make her pregnancy easier by any means possible.

Find out things she has to deal with in her everyday life that you can take off her hands, even if it means a little extra effort on your part. Be considerate of things she can no longer do all the time. If she's having trouble with morning sickness, keep crackers and ginger ale in all parts of the house. Finally, let her know you love her. Plan a good old-fashioned date night, complete with flowers and some well-thought-out plans. It might be a fun time to relive some of those old memories.

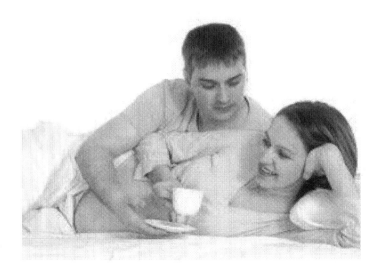

HANDLING THE HORMONES

I hate to stereotype, but it requires so much less thought. So, if the following description doesn't jibe with your experience, I apologize in advance. The implantation of the egg into the uterus causes the production of hCG (or beta hCG), the pregnancy hormone. It causes the production of estrogen and progesterone. These hormones are quite necessary for the development of the baby, but like steroids and unprotected sex, they have side effects. As production of the hormones continues, the levels in her body begin to increase. During weeks 5, 6, and 7, pregnancy hormones start making your BMP crazy. Like DEFCON 1 crazy. Typical symptoms include nausea, fatigue, and tender nipples, plus urinating more than your grandfather.

YOU VERSUS THE HORMONES

You versus the hormones is like Spinks versus Tyson, Joe versus the volcano, and Tiger versus monogamy. You have no chance. The pregnancy hormones are just too high. They make her emotions change, and they make her body change. Lots of regular foods she used to enjoy might make her react as if you just cut loose some mighty Taco Bell- driven wind. Her moods may become as unpredictable as a roulette wheel, and you'll have similar odds at predicting them. Fatigue becomes a major issue and her bedtime and dinnertime may start to coincide with one another. But on a positive note, her all-day sickness (we're starting a campaign to rename "morning sickness") may show some signs of slowing down, although for many women it rages on into the second trimester before subsiding. Constipation and flatulence, gifts from your unborn angel, may become significant at these times. Just pretend you're back in freshman year of college with a roommate who has rapidly gained weight, farts all the time, and sleeps a lot. But there is one significant difference. The extra bra size she has gained has you thinking this pregnancy may have some benefits after all.

CHORES, DADDY STYLE

In the beginning, you were just so glad to be pregnant. As your little science project grew, your BMP began to wear down, up to the point where if she was eating at all, she was elbowing seniors out of the way at their favorite Early Bird Special spot so she could get to bed by 6pm.

Men, in general, show support and affection by providing financially for their families. These people may attempt to help by bringing in cleaning services to knock out those things called chores. But women don't always take kindly to having strangers invade their home. Besides, many times you have these invasive (and expensive) visitors come in to clean only to find they have done everything wrong in the eyes of your significant other. The best, but most unattractive, the solution may be to show support with your actions, even if this includes scrubbing toilets and doing the laundry.

Of all the changes Junior will bring to your schedule, social life, financial life, and sex life, it's the physical changes to your BMP that are starting to be most evident now. Quite a few changes are going on, both inside and out. Let's take a moment to consider some of them. Yes, Sparky, I know: breast enlargement is one of them.

1. Belly. Somewhere around week 12, the baby begins to pooch out. Between months 2 and 3, her uterus will have grown to her belly button. By the end of the whole shooting match, that

little miracle will have stretched things out up toward her rib cage.

2. Breasts. I will attempt to keep this section purely as it pertains to the gestation of your future child. Her breasts are preparing to produce milk for the baby. Estrogen, among other hormones, is working to increase the glands that produce this nutritious liquid. During pregnancy, these changes can often lead to breast enlargement (see, I'm biting my tongue). Her breasts may feel slightly firm and are often tender trying to hold back. Your partner may need a bigger bra as this growth progresses. Oh, for God's sake, let the puppies breathe!

3. Heart. Okay, I'm back. Sorry for that unnecessary outburst. Because of the future child taking up residence in Hotel Uterus, your BMP's blood supply will increase by one-third to one-half by the end of her pregnancy. In turn, her heart has to work harder to move this blood around. Her heartbeat can change from a usual resting rate of about 70 beats per minute to a comfortable pace of between 80 to 90 beats per minute. Keep this in mind when you're out for your daily twenty-miler with your BMP. She may not be able to keep up with her usual pace.

4. Gastrointestinal system. Those good old hormones are at it again. Some of the same hormones vital to maintaining a healthy pregnancy can also cause nausea and vomiting, along with other GI problems. If the breast enlargement section got you all hot and bothered, here's the antidote: belching, constipation, and increased flatulence are common during pregnancy. How's that for a cold shower?

5. Skin. The ever-present hormones can cause her skin to show brown patches as additional melanin is produced. There is even individual rashes only pregnant women experience.

So, love her body, whatever the shape or size. Encourage her. Touch her with familiarity, whether it's with a gentle neck rub or holding her hand at the mall. The bottom line is that you want to communicate to her your feelings for her haven't changed or wavered no matter what her shape is in at the moment. All you can hope for is that she'll return the favor as you slowly lose your figure, hair, and all sense of style.

MANAGING WEIGHT GAIN

Your BMP is going to gain weight. Another human is trapped in there, after all. So, there's some truth to the saying that she's eating for two. But you, on the other hand, are not, so don't act like it. Whether you're eating for one or two, all bodies prefer a healthy diet to a steady stream of chicken wings.

You may be picturing her being all healthy while you continue to plow through a plate of cheese fries. I don't recommend it. It would feel like watching your friends accidentally stumble into a free all-you-can-drink event sponsored by the Swedish Bikini All-Stars on the night you're the designated driver. So, be considerate and behave around her. Moderation in your drinking, especially if it was something she enjoyed before pregnancy, is the prudent course. If the impregnation magic happened after a night of partying, don't pull out the "it reminds me of our night together and our child's conception" speech. She ain't buying it, no matter how great your sales skills. Playing the game this way may even earn you a couple of guilt-free nights out with your BMP's blessing. The key word is **might**.

As for smokes, give them up. It's for your good — and your baby's. Secondhand smoke will have your child sounding like a truck driver and rebuilding carburetors before his or her third birthday, not to mention all the other health conditions it can cause or worsen.

As your BMP gains weight with the growth of your seed, you may also gain weight. Don't give us the research about "sympathy weight." Do something good for yourself and eat healthfully with her.

PICKLES AND ICE CREAM

If you watch enough movies, you'll see a poor father-to-be sent out in the middle of the night because his pregnant wife craves something. You've seen it before, right? The clock shows 2am., and she shakes the poor boy awake. Invariably, she tells him that he needs to run to the store right now for some bizarre combination of foods. The guy, of course, simply cannot say no to her because she's pregnant. Much humor ensues.

It's true. Many report that their BMPs craved food from a particular restaurant. Some claim their partners wanted salty foods, while others say it was an ice cream sundae that was in such demand. The medical field hasn't conclusively documented the reasons for these stereotypical cravings. Their theories remain just that. As any man who has been through the process will tell you, it's probably best just to get her what she wants, when she wants it, if humanly possible.

Despite the hype, I've never been asked to run to the store at midnight for pickles and ice cream. Except for that one time in college but nobody was pregnant.

PREGNANCY MASSAGE

It's time for the two of you to reconnect. I understand that your secret weapon is the art of seductive massage. I further understand that taking this weapon of mass seduction away from you is like sending a gladiator into the ring without his sword. But alas, I need to de-sword you. Don't try to play amateur masseur here. Incorrect message can trigger contractions. Aromatherapy can also cause problems. Find a massage therapist who is specially trained in massaging pregnant women and give your BMP a gift certificate.

Or better still, take the time to learn what messages you can safely give (ask her doctor). With all the remodeling going on, she's likely to be sore. By likely, I mean 100 percent of pregnant women report feeling this way. Besides, what better way for you two to relax together?

PREGNANCY SEX

Having sex once she's pregnant is overkill. Just kidding! It's not as easy as it was, though. Between your feeling strange about the whole "sex while pregnant" situation and everything she's got going on in there, it can get quite complicated when it comes to celebrating your love with your lover.

Depending on your luck, your BMP won't look any different for three or four months; and during months four through six, if you blink fast you can convince yourself she still doesn't look any different. With your doctor's assurance in hand that you can't hurt the baby (please direct questions about this issue to your doctor), you can let your strong instincts take over. Now it's business as usual in the bedroom and without worries about getting her pregnant because you're already there!

But at some point, there's no denying it: she's pregnant and you can tell. As for the prospect of having relations with a pregnant woman, I say you go all in. Presumably, you love this person, and as long as your doc gives you the thumbs-up, it's all good. Don't underestimate the fact that once the little angel has arrived, you'll be exhausted for the next twelve months or more, and the energy you used to put into planning a sexy rendezvous will be gone. Instead of spending your free time on frivolous things like your hobbies and the laundry, your waking moments will be consumed with thoughts of a nap. Nap in the car, nap in the afternoon, spot-nap on the Burger King counter while waiting for order #123. Once that bundle of joy and tears arrives, you will take sleep wherever and whenever you can get it. By now you should be starting to get the point. Your sex life, among other things, will be drastically affected, and you two need to enjoy each other while your time and energy permits.

EXERCISE DURING PREGNANCY

Let's face it. In today's world of fifty-hour workweeks and long commutes, we all need some training. But it's especially important for your BMP to get regular exercise during her pregnancy. What are the benefits? More energy, sounder sleep, increased muscle strength, and reduction of various pregnancy symptoms, as well as the benefit of bouncing back into shape faster post-pregnancy than if she doesn't exercise.

If she's already exercising regularly, she'll probably be able to continue her routine. Of course, all training programs need to be cleared with her doctor first. If she isn't already active, it's unlikely that she'll be encouraged to start an intensive exercise program; but mild exercise, like walking can still benefit your BMP. Pregnant women may also benefit from yoga classes specifically targeted toward them. Don't miss the opportunity to skip working out your already perfect pectorals to do a workout with her. She will appreciate the support, I promise! (Did I mention that you need to consult your real doctor first?)

Here's a wild idea: if you aren't exercising already, why don't you do the same? It can only help people on the street be able to tell definitively which one of you is pregnant.

MATERNITY CLOTHES

Forget your dog; maternity clothes are a man's best friend. What doesn't man love special shopping trips where you purchase clothes you know for a fact will only be good for a few months? Adding to the fun is the fact that many maternity clothing stores are very proud of their clothes. You can tell by the amount they overcharge you.

The good news is that you now have evidence that she wasn't just faking it for the last few months to turn you into her slave. Now the bad news: she's going to need a whole new wardrobe. If you're lucky, you can beg, borrow or steal what salvageable "gently used" maternity clothes you can from friends and family to minimize the financial impact. Otherwise, you're going to spend a mortgage payment on clothes. One more tip: if she asks your opinion when trying on clothes, be neutral.

One more tip: if she asks your opinion when trying on clothes, be neutral. A quick note, though: don't get rid of these clothes if you plan to have more children, or if you intend to have unprotected sex without birth control. Nothing would be more of a double dose of fun than an unplanned pregnancy, plus a maternity clothes shopping spree after you'd just gotten rid of her last maternity wardrobe.

So now we know that caring for a pregnant woman is more complicated than we first thought. Thanks to the pregnancy hormones, her mood, and her needs are a moving target. These are the times where you can score some major points by helping take care of her and easing the difficulties of pregnancy in any way possible. In addition to caring for her physically, don't forget to show her that you love the curves. Compliments and gentle, doctor-approved massages are an excellent way to do this.

CHAPTER 10: HEALING YOUR VAGINA NATURALLY

During pregnancy, many women experience swelling, discharge, varicosities (veins popping out), and other symptoms that affect the vagina. Your vagina is sore, swollen, and in serious need of some TLC. Following vaginal birth, pain, swelling, bleeding, and overall discomfort is par for the course.

The time it will take for your vaginal tissue to heal and recover is variable depending on the extent of the trauma—including if you had a tear or episiotomy. Caring for your body using natural remedies will not only help you recover more quickly but will also decrease the amount of discomfort you are experiencing.

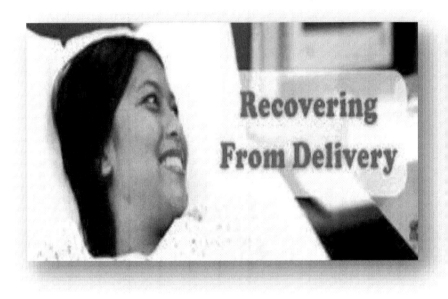

EARLY VAGINAL BLEEDING

Lochia is the medical term for the vaginal bleeding that occurs postpartum. It is normal, and you will often see many clots, which can vary in size. The bleeding transitions from red to brown and eventually becomes a yellow or clear discharge. For many women, the release will be gone by four weeks postpartum, but some may have discharge up to 8 weeks.

If you experience a new onset of heavy bleeding or large clots after the discharge has stopped or feel concerned about the release, be sure to speak with your healthcare provider.

Do not use a tampon, menstrual cup or insert anything into the vagina during your first six weeks postpartum. Instead, opt for organic pads and often change to avoid vaginal irritation.

NATURAL REMEDIES TO HEAL AND SOOTHE SORE TISSUE

Sitz Baths. Traditional sits baths, which consist of having one tub with cold water and another with warm that you alternate between, are the most ideal, but you may not have easy access to a bathtub or even have the energy to set up a sitz bath. Because of this, I recommend a modified postpartum sitz bath utilizing herbs to encourage tissue healing and soothe the area.

Postpartum sitz bath. Place the herbs directly into a muslin bag and immerse the bag in the hot water of the bath. To do this, run the bath water with only hot water, place the muslin bag and one cup of Epsom salt into the tub water and allow to steep. Once the water has reached a comfortable temperature, you can get into the bathtub. Remember, you only need enough to cover the genital area, so if you're not up for a full bath, just place a small amount of water in the bathtub.

Herbs for Sitz Baths

- Calendula flower: antimicrobial, soothing, anti-inflammatory
- Rosemary leaves: antimicrobial
- Comfrey leaves: promotes tissue healing
- Lavender flower: antimicrobial, relaxing
- Thyme leaves: antimicrobial
- Uva ursi berry: antimicrobial
- Shepherd's purse leaf: hemostatic (stops blood flow)
- Yarrow: antibacterial, antifungal, hemostatic

Choose ½ cup each of four to six of these herbs and place in a large bowl to mix well. Place the herbs in a large Mason jar and store in a cool, dry place. When ready to use, take ¼ cup of the mixture and place in a muslin bag for your bath or use any of the following methods.

It's important that you do not apply too much heat or stay immersed in hot water for too long as it can create pelvic stagnation. Consider ending the bath after 20 minutes of heat or when the water cools.

To increase circulation and promote healing, and the bath with a cold compress placed directly on the genital area for 10 minutes or run cool water over the vaginal tissue for 30 seconds.

Making a Topical Tea. Bring two quarts of water to a boil. Add one cup of herbs and remove from the heat. Cover and allow to sit for 20 minutes. Strain and allow to cool. Use as a rinse at the end of your shower.

Note: The herbal mixture will keep at room temperature for about 6-8 hours, in the fridge for three days. Do not take internally.

Herbal Peri Bottle Rinse. Place cooled Topical Tea (see above) in a peri bottle. To use, apply a stream of fluid from the peri bottle to the vaginal tissue during urination and following using the restroom.

Herbal Cold Compresses. Apply the Topical Tea to organic pads or reusable organic cloth and place in the freezer. Use these cold packs to the vaginal tissue, either allowing them to warm or removing after 10-15 minutes. Take care not to over-apply cold compresses.

Apply as often as you find necessary for the first three to seven days.

What if I'm birthing in a hospital?

You can make individual muslin herb bags before delivery and store them in plastic bags or storage containers to keep in your hospital bag. In a pinch, you can place them in a basin of boiling water and use both the water and muslin herb bag to cleanse the area once the water has reached a comfortable temperature.

WHEN TO TALK TO YOUR HEALTHCARE PROVIDER:

If you've had a major tear, trauma, or an infection, please discuss these therapies with your doctor. They may be contraindicated in early postpartum. Signs of infection include fever, chills, nausea, vomiting, extreme redness, tenderness, foul odor, or pus.

HEALING VAGINAL TEARS & EPISIOTOMY

If you've experienced severe tearing, ask your doctor about using a limited antimicrobial following bowel movements and urination. Sometimes, a simple water and iodine solution will be recommended if you don't have an iodine allergy

Keeping a clean peri bottle next to the sink to be used when you void will help decrease discomfort. Fill it with warm water and express the water onto the urethra during urination to help dilute the urine to make the sensitive tissue more comfortable. You can also use the herbal sitz baths wash solution in the peri bottle.

Using the same principles and techniques to heal the vaginal tissue as previously discussed will also improve the healing of tears. Some women have residual pain and discomfort even after the tissue has healed. If this is the case for you, you should consider speaking with your doctor and a pelvic floor physical therapist.

In my practice, I've helped many women to resolve scar tissue and restore their tissue integrity, as well as create more uniform tone.

HEALING VULVOVAGINAL VARICOSITIES (DILATED VEINS)

During pregnancy, there is lots of pressure on the pelvis and, as a result, circulation isn't at its best. Many women experience mild dilations of the veins in the vulvar area. It is not uncommon for these to resolve after pregnancy; however, if they become enlarged, hot, or painful after birth, please speak with your doctor.

Sitz Baths. Sitz baths using comfrey, yellow dock, plantain, and yarrow reduce swelling and relieve discomfort.

Hydrotherapy. Alternating hot and cold hydrotherapy heals the tissue and increases circulation. For new moms, I recommend performing hydrotherapy in the shower. At the end of your shower, turn the water to cool-cold and apply directly to your pelvis and the affected area. If you have a removable shower head, use the cold water directly to the veins.

Apply warm water for 1 minute followed by cold water for 30 seconds. Repeat for a total of 3 rounds, always ending with cold.

Vitamin E. 400 IU daily, taken internally to promote antioxidant activity and healing of the blood vessels may be used. You may also apply the oil topically to the affected tissue to soothe and aid in healing.

Bioflavonoids. 1,000 mg. daily supports blood vessel integrity to prevent the vein from enlarging further.

Homeopathic Calc Fluor cell salt 6x. 3-5 tabs three times daily to stabilize connective tissue.

ORGAN PROLAPSE

I recommend that women rest in bed and lay down as often as possible for at least two weeks following childbirth. Relaxin, the hormone that allowed your cervix to soften and your hips to widen, can remain in your system up to 6 months after delivery. Therefore, some women experience joint instability and can be injured with new intense exercise.

Why is it important to minimize time on your feet? In the beginning, when relaxing is still high, the uterus is bulky, and the pelvic floor muscles are in need of recovery, you are at risk for developing a vaginal and uterine prolapse. The combination of all these factors, plus gravity and the potential overextending yourself can put you at even greater risk. Refrain from being overly active is the main message I want you to walk away with. Yes, you can grab a snack, use the restroom and engage in a very light activity, but in those early weeks focus on resting as often as possible.

In Chinese medicine, they recommend that the feet don't touch the floor for the first 40 days following childbirth. It is a beautiful illustration of the kind of support you'll need in those first weeks after giving birth. Obviously, this is ideal but not always possible.

If you don't have a lot of support and you feel that you need to be on your feet and taking care of things, try taking frequent breaks.

Some of my patients have found it helpful to set a timer so that they aren't standing for longer than 20 minutes at a time. If you feel heaviness begin to develop in your pelvis, take this as a sign that it is time to rest. Sensations of pressure and bulging are familiar with pelvic prolapse.

TYPES OF PROLAPSE:

Cystocele (Anterior Vaginal Wall Prolapse): Herniation of the anterior wall (belly button side) of the vagina, with or without dropping of the bladder.

Common Symptoms: Urinary incontinence or difficulty with urination.

Rectocele (Posterior Vaginal Wall Prolapse): Herniation of the posterior wall (back side) of the vagina, with or without dropping of the rectum.

Common Symptoms: Constipation, fecal incontinence, urgency.

Enterocele: Intestines protrude through or to the vaginal wall.

Common Symptoms: Pelvic fullness, pelvic pain, bulge sensation in the vagina, pain with intercourse, pulling sensation in the pelvis that is better with lying down.

Apical Compartment Prolapse: Descent of the uterus or upper portion of the vagina to the opening of the vagina.

Common Symptoms: Urinary incontinence or difficulty with urination, bulge sensation in the vagina.

Because the vagina is a continuous organ, it can be difficult to differentiate a prolapse and often there can be an issue with several aspects of the vagina.

Working with a skilled pelvic floor provider to rehabilitate stretched muscles and support the organs of the pelvis will enable your body to heal. Further medical intervention may be necessary, and your health care provider can assist you in ensuring you have the necessary care to heal your body.

VAGINAL WIND

Vaginal wind or the release of air from the vagina is widespread in the early postpartum healing. There's a lot of laxity in the tissue. You passed a human through a minimal space—which has weakened your vaginal tone. While it can feel embarrassing, it's nothing to be ashamed of. It's very common. Most women experience it.

Performing Kegels can help you regain tone. You may also consider working with a trained pelvic floor professional to increase your vaginal tone.

Because many women feel embarrassed when there is a release of air from the vagina, you may want to practice exercises or yoga moves at home before you go to class. For example, audible vaginal gas can be passed when moving from down dog (a yoga pose) into another position, and although completely healthy it is far from ideal.

IS A 6-WEEK CHECKUP NECESSARY?

You should have your 6-week check up with your doctor or midwife following delivery. It is where they check how the tissue is repairing and healing, making sure that there are no signs of infection and that your uterus is healing properly. It's more than just getting clearance for sex and exercise. While it's important to know whether your body is ready for these activities, it's also important to have other symptoms evaluated at that time.

LABS TO CONSIDER TESTING POSTPARTUM

Depending on what your birth was like, your current symptoms, good history and family history your doctor may want to order labs anywhere from 6 weeks to 3 months postpartum.

Lab	Evaluation
Complete Blood Count (CBC)	Evaluates white blood cells, red blood cells, and screen for anemia.
Ferritin	Evaluates iron stores.
Comprehensive Metabolic Panel (CMP)	Evaluates liver, kidney, and gallbladder function.
Thyroid Panel (TSH, Total T3, Total T4, Free T3, Free T4, Reverse T3)	Evaluates thyroid function and health.
Thyroid Antibodies (Anti-TPO,	Screens for autoimmune postpartum

Anti-Thyroglobulin)	thyroiditis.
Vitamin D	Determine vitamin D status and evaluate if supplementation is warranted.
B12 and Methylmalonic Acid	Evaluates vitamin B12 status.
Folate	Evaluates folate status.
Homocysteine	An indirect marker of inflammation that also gives insight into B vitamin utilization.
MTHFR Gene	Evaluate if there are underlying genetic issues that may affect mental health, energy use and detox pathways.
HgA1C	Marker of blood sugar over a 3-month period. Important if you had gestational diabetes.
CRP and ESR	Measurement of inflammation
Salivary Cortisol	Determines function and health of adrenal glands.

NATURAL RELIEF FOR AFTER BIRTH PAINS

After birth pains are normal and they can be pretty extreme for some women. They are the result of your uterus contracting back to its original size, a process known as involution.

These contractions begin about 12 hours following delivery and may be as mild as your menstrual cramps or as intense as labor contractions. Each time you nurse in the early days following birth, you will also feel these contractions. This is because baby's nursing stimulates the release of oxytocin, often called the "cuddle hormone," which causes contractions and helped return your uterus to its original size, among other things. Another benefit to breastfeeding!

In addition to returning your uterus to its original size, these contractions also prevent excess bleeding, which is why it is important to avoid aspirin. Aspirin thins the blood and can lead to increased bleeding.

If you feel like you need to take something for these contractions, try to avoid acetaminophen or ibuprofen as these have side effects that can impact your health, such as leading to intestinal irritation. Instead, keep the following remedies near you when you breastfeed to alleviate pain:

Homeopathic Mag Phots 6C. Take 3-5 pellets every 15 minutes for pain. You may find it helpful to take a dose just before you begin nursing.

Hot Water Bottle. Apply heat up to 20 minutes to the small abdomen. Wrap the outside of the hot water bottle with a towel and avoid making contact with baby.

Cramp Bark (Viburnum opulus) Tincture. Take two droppers full just before you nurse. It reduces pain without inhibiting the uterus from shrinking.

Motherwort (Leonurus cardiac) Tincture. Take two droppers full up to 4 times daily. Motherwort is a uterine tonic that eases anxiety, irritability, and supports a healthy heart.

Uterine Massage. Every time before you stand up for the first 3-6 weeks postpartum, massage your uterus. Make your hand into a fist and knead the lower belly. This is a technique that may help decrease the amount of bleeding and helps the uterus heal.

NATURAL REMEDIES TO HEAL URINARY TRACT INFECTIONS

Urgency, frequency, or pain with urination may be a sign of a urinary tract infection (UTI). It is wise to contact your doctor if you experience these symptoms, especially if you have a fever, nausea, back ache, or see blood in your urine. If caught early you may not require an antibiotic. However, if there is any risk of the infection affecting your kidneys you want to act quickly and meet with your doctor, as an antibiotic will be necessary to resolve the infection and protect your kidneys.

Prevention:

- Wear white cotton underwear changed daily
- Use only mild, natural detergents on clothing
- Use non-deodorized, preferably organic, sanitary pads
- Wipe front to back after bowel movement
- Avoid bubble baths
- Shower after swimming
- Avoid tight pants
- Eat Lacto-fermented foods three times weekly

Natural Treatment of Urinary Tract Infection

Diet:

Avoid sugar, alcohol, caffeine, aspartame, and dried fruits until symptoms resolve.

Increase Water Intake: Drink a glass of filtered water every 20 minutes for 2 hours then every hour for 24 hours, except during sleep.

Vitamin C: 1,000 mg 4-5 times daily for two days. Can cause loose stools, so decrease the dose if this occurs. After two days, reduce dose to 500 mg 4-5 times daily for five days.

Cranberry Juice: Drink 4 ounces of unsweetened cranberry juice four times daily for one week.

Cranberry D-Mannose: 2 capsules twice daily for one week.

Homeopathic Remedies:

- Cantharis 30C: Use when there is painful burning with urination.
- Equisetum 30C: Use when there is pain, and there's a sensation that the bladder is always full, despite having just urinated.
- Sarsparilla 30C: Pain at the end of urination, may not be able to void unless done so standing up.
- Berberis 30C: Painful bladder, relieved by urination.
- Staphysagria 30C: UTI comes on after intercourse.

To use Homeopathic remedies: 3-5 pellets 15-minutes away from food every 2-4 hours until symptoms are resolved.

URINARY INCONTINENCE

You sneeze, you see. You a cough, you pee. You pick up your baby and you pee. It is not only inconvenient but also embarrassing. And it's also a common symptom following childbirth.

Some women will easily recover and will not experience long-term issues with urination, while others will go on to experience a daily incontinence or urinary leakage.

NATURAL HEALING AFTER A C-SECTION

I think it is important to acknowledge that there is no shame in having a C-section. Many women, especially those who were planning a natural birth, feel ashamed and sometimes defeated after a C-section as if they did something wrong because they didn't deliver their baby vaginally. There is no shame in doing whatever it took to bring your child into this world and to ensure their health and yours, no matter the procedure.

Regardless of the type of delivery, you are a mother, and you have a beautiful baby to be grateful for. You 'reincredible—today and every day.

For most women, a small layer of skin begins to heal the wound within 48 hours, protecting it from bacterial infections. However, this skin is fragile and easily disrupted. Typically, women can shower after the first 48 hours following delivery.

Please contact your health care provider immediately if you experience pain at the site, fever, discharge from the wound, the tissue becomes red, or there is an odor present.

Many women find the following tips helpful in healing from a C-Section.

Keep the wound dry and clean. After your showers, gently pat the wound area dry. Avoid clothing, which rubs against the wound site.

Bone Broth. Drink at least one cup daily. Along with being easy to digest, bone broth is rich in minerals and amino acids to aid your body in healing. **See recipe**.

Grass-fed Gelatin. Consume 2-4 tablespoons daily. Another source of amino acids to support connective tissue healing.

Rest and Sleep. You are recovering from surgery. Take it slow and allow your body time to heal.

Ask for Help. Get help wherever you can to reduce the need to be up and about.

Anything you can get help with to reduce your need to be up and about will allow your body the much-needed time it needs to rest.

Healing Herbal Wash

This green wash is antimicrobial, which prevents infections and keeps the area clean. The comfrey and calendula promote rapid tissue healing and healthy skin.

- 2 ounces comfrey leaves
- 2 ounces calendula flowers

- Two tablespoons Oregon grape root
- 1-ounce lavender flowers
- One tablespoon sea salt

Mix the herbs in a large bowl. Bring 1 gallon (4 quarts) of water to a boil in a large pot. Turn off heat and add one large handful of herbs to the pot and stir. Cover the mixture for overnight, strain the herbs and store the liquid in the fridge. It will keep for three days.

When you're ready to use, place sea salt in a peri bottle and fill the bottle with the herbal liquid. Shake well.

In the shower, use the herbal wash to cleanse the wound area gently.

You can use this green wash daily. In my house, I keep calendula flowers and Oregon grape root on hand to make a quick wound care wash for when my little one gets a scrape.

CONCLUSION

Pregnancy is an exciting journey, and you are probably more prepared than you realize. If not, this book will provide you with facts around 'what to expect when you are expecting.'

Therefore 'before gives birth.' You may also hear health professionals use the term gestation. This is the period or process, from conception to birth, of the baby developing in the womb.

It is because every time you have a period your body is preparing for pregnancy. It also serves as a gauge for health professionals, as it's hard for them to know precisely when conception occurred. Your expected delivery date is therefore calculated 40 weeks and from the first day of your last period. Thank you for downloading this book I hope you will apply the acquired knowledge productively.

Lastly, if you really enjoyed reading the book, I would like to kindly ask you to take time out to share your insights by posting a review on Amazon. It'd be really appreciated.

Made in the USA
San Bernardino, CA
01 May 2018